A Resource Guide for Doctors, Nurses, and Technologists

Patient Sedation Without Medication

Rapid rapport and quick hypnotic techniques

By Elvira Lang, MD and Eleanor Laser, PhD

Published 2009.

14 13 12 11 10 09   1 2 3 4 5

Printed in the United States of America

Design: DECODE, Inc., Seattle

What Professionals Are Saying About *Patient Sedation Without Medication*

"Patient Sedation Without Medication *is a book for every medical practitioner who wants to provide optimal patient comfort and reduce procedure time. It is sure to be a classic.*"

—Arreed Barabasz, PhD, Editor of the International Journal of Clinical and Experimental Hypnosis, Author of *Hypnotherapeutic Techniques 2E*

"*My using the techniques detailed in* Patient Sedation Without Medication *throughout radiology procedures has improved the experience for my patients as well as myself. I have had one patient ask, 'When will we be starting?' only to tell him, 'We are done!'*"

—William Barnhart, Radiology Technologist, Iowa City, Iowa

"*Frankly, I was a skeptic about procedure hypnosis until my own patients experienced successful interventions by Dr. Lang and her team utilizing the techniques described in* Patient Sedation Without Medication. *It really works! This book will be an outstanding resource for clinicians involved with procedures that otherwise would require sedation.*"

—Paul A. Church, MD, Urology Practice Associates, Boston, MA

"*I have been performing interventional radiology procedures for forty years and have worked with Dr. Lang for the past decade. Her hypnosis techniques—made easily accessible for the reader in* Patient Sedation Without Medication*—are especially helpful with difficult patients. It is impressive to see how the overall tension in the suite dissipates once the technologist or nurse begins the hypnosis.*"

—Melvin Clouse, MD, BIDMC, Vice Chairman Emeritus, Deaconess Professor of Radiology, Harvard Medical School

"*How wonderful to discover a medical book—*Patient Sedation Without Medication*—that is not only engaging to read, but offers life lessons that can be used by anyone in or out of the medical profession.*"

—Daryn Eller, Health Writer for *Ladies Home Journal, Prevention, Parents,* and other national publications

"*Dr. Lang is a modern medical pioneer. In* Patient Sedation Without Medication, *she and Dr. Laser share how to apply their techniques during medical procedures. This book—based on solid science, good clinical wisdom, and common sense—will become the bible of patient care. Every physician, nurse, and medical technologist who reads it and absorbs its lessons will become a more humane and effective caregiver.*"

—Bruce N. Eimer, PhD, ABPP, Clinical Psychologist, Author of ***Hypnotize Yourself Out of Pain Now!***, Co-author of ***Brief Cognitive Hypnosis, Pain Management Psychotherapy: A Practical Guide***

"*Dr. Lang's group has documented that hypnotic techniques expedite and simplify surgical procedures and has also quantitated the time and money saved. As our national debate continues to revolve around lowering cost, while improving patient comfort and satisfaction,* Patient Sedation Without Medication *will be a beacon for all who do these exacting procedures.*"

—Dabney M. Ewin, MD, FACS, Clinical Professor of Surgery and Psychiatry, Universities of Tulane and Louisiana, New Orleans

"*Lang and Laser really get it: patients' fears, their helplessness when caught in the midst of medical procedures, and the huge need of patients to be treated with dignity and respect.*"

—Judy Foreman, Nationally Syndicated Health Columnist

"Patient Sedation Without Medication *is a wonderful work that provides the clinician with specific 'how to' information for helping patients achieve comfort during medical procedures. Any healthcare provider wanting to help his or her patients be more comfortable would enjoy reading this book and applying the effective strategies that are so clearly described.*"

—Mark P. Jensen, PhD, Professor and Vice Chair for Research, Department of Rehabilitation Medicine, University of Washington

"Patient Sedation Without Medication *provides a comprehensive guide to the use of hypnosis in a medical setting. It presents complex information in clear and concise manner and is a wonderful resource to the practicing clinician and the clinical educator.*"

—Kate Kravits, RN, MA, LPC, ATR-BC, HNB-BC, Senior Research Specialist, City of Hope, Duarte, California

"With a keen intellect and a compassionate heart, the authors have provided a roadmap to effectively implement rapid hypnotic techniques into the everyday practice of medicine—a brilliant job of translating scientific work into a formula readily accessible by any busy medical team."

—Henrietta L. Logan, PhD, Professor and Director Southeast Center for Research to Reduce Disparities in Oral Health, University of Florida

"Procedure hypnosis—as refined by Dr. Lang—allows patients to self-regulate pain, anxiety, and discomfort both in preparation of and during surgical and diagnostic procedures. The result: in the procedural suite, there is ONE TEAM working together to alleviate suffering. Patient Sedation Without Medication *explains how!"*

—Sylvain Néron, PhD, Louise Granofsky Psychosocial Oncology Program, Segal Cancer Center—Jewish General Hospital, Montréal, PQ Canada

"Dr. Lang is the foremost authority in the world on procedure hypnosis. She and her team have developed and rigorously studied techniques that help patients achieve the greatest possible control of pain and anxiety. Patient Sedation Without Medication *is the premier knowledge base for these powerful and effective techniques."*

—Max Shapiro, MD, Director of Education and Research of the New England Society of Hypnosis (NESH)

"Patient Sedation Without Medication *provides a lucid description of painless ways to provide effective and humane support to patients undergoing stressful medical procedures. In this book, hypnosis, the oldest form of psychotherapy, becomes the most modern of medical tools to help patients restructure their perception and experience. Read it and use it—your patients will thank you."*

—David Spiegel, MD, Willson Professor and Associate Chair Psychiatry & Behavioral Sciences, Stanford University School of Medicine, Co-author of *Trance and Treatment: Clinical Uses of Hypnosis*

"Using the straightforward and effective methods in Patient Sedation Without Medication, *the caregivers in the office can reduce patient pain and facilitate treatment dramatically."*

—Dr. Chris Tomshack, Founder and CEO of HealthSource Chiropractic and Progressive Rehab

Contents

Cases

Journal Entries

Introduction

I wish I had had a book like *Patient Sedation Without Medication* when I started my career as an interventional radiologist performing surgeries on patients who were awake. Faced with procedure risks and patients' distress, I was often struggling with the same question: "How can I get this patient safely and comfortably through this medical encounter?" I wished for a magic wand that could dissipate the stress, anxiety, and pain that I was witnessing everyday. Yes, there were drugs—but drugs are no magic wand—they come with limits and carry their own medical risks. I saw time after time how patients' fears could easily override even massive doses of sedatives. Moreover, the increased doses, unfortunately, kicked in with full power when the procedure was over; and the delayed effect greatly complicated recovery. I wanted something that would render practitioners capable of helping in a way that would add to rather than take away from the patient's sense of personal resourcefulness and effectiveness. Something that would return them from the procedure alert and ready to heal rather than "knocked out."

About 17 years ago, at the Veterans Affairs Medical Center in Palo Alto, California, I watched a very scared Vietnam Veteran go calmly though a medical procedure that he, before now, always faced with the expression of horrific fears. The calming force that changed his experience from terror to calm was hypnotic imagery. Here, I thought, just might be that magic wand. As a pragmatist I was excited, but as a scientist and physician I was also cautious. I wanted to make sure that hypnosis would be effective for a broad range of patients and feasible in a modern, rushed, often hectic, medical environment. Thus I started an intensive research program with federal funding.

A few years later, after my move to direct the Interventional Radiology Division at the University of Iowa Hospitals and Clinics in 1995, I searched for an experienced hypnotherapist to help me train my new team. I had the good fortune to find Dr. Laser and we have been collaborating ever since.

I was pleasantly surprised to get the call from Dr. Lang requesting that I travel to the University of Iowa Hospital and Clinics to conduct training in procedure hypnosis for her radiology team. I've long been convinced of the potential of hypnosis in healthcare. My father, an obstetrician, had begun to study hypnosis and utilize it in his practice before his untimely death. He saw great potential in the use of hypnosis in the medical setting and shared his interest with me, which inspired me to pursue it. I was further inspired to explore the possibilities of procedure hypnosis by the tragic loss of my mother whose death during surgery was attributed to anesthesia.

When Dr. Lang called, I was specializing in hypnotherapy in my psychology practice and I was already, as people say, "on board." Perhaps that is why I was surprised to find that not everyone in the group I was to train was optimistic. Hypnosis in the hospital was a new idea to the nurses and technicians and several seemed unsure of the process and unsure of their ability to learn it. With Dr. Lang there to ease the way, I began to work on both concerns. I was determined to help these professionals see the advantage and gain the confidence they needed to incorporate a package of rapport and quick hypnotic techniques to connect with patients and to bring them relief. My training focus was limited to the set of quick-to-learn/quick-to-apply skills appropriate to the radiological suite. It turned out to be a mutual learning experience. I helped them realize that the techniques are easy and very effective. My application ideas were opened to new heights when Dr. Lang gave me my first opportunity to practice these skills in an operating theater. The experience gave me insight into ways I could nuance my approach. My time working with these professionals inspired me to join Dr. Lang's efforts and to do what I could to ensure that nurses, technicians, and other licensed healthcare professionals were awakened to the potential of hypnosis, were trained to use hypnotic techniques appropriate for their situations, and were officially accepted by professional societies to include the practice of hypnosis within their professional duties. The realization of the importance of training of these professional groups lead to bylaw changes first within the New England Society of Clinical Hypnosis, then the Society of Clinical and Experimental Hypnosis, and most recently the American Society of Clinical Hypnosis.

Our goal in writing *Patient Sedation Without Medication* is to share with all healthcare professionals the fruits of our research and of our experience with procedure hypnosis. In this book we have compiled what we learned over the years from helping patients through procedures, diagnostic examinations, and medical encounters. We tested the rapid rapport and quick hypnotic techniques presented in this book in rigorous prospective randomized studies with >700 patients. Our studies clearly showed that the use of rapid rapport and quick hypnotic techniques made procedures more comfortable, safer, and faster.

Our research was conducted in the field; every technique was tested in the fire of busy medical practices in hospitals and private practice settings. Over the years, we have clarified our presentations to learners and refined the methods and techniques. What we have distilled from our efforts is a set of rapid rapport and quick hypnotic techniques that healthcare professionals can easily learn and readily incorporate into their unique professional daily work duties. In this book, we tell you what worked well for us—and what didn't. You don't have to start from scratch, and you can avoid our missteps.

The subject of this book is procedure hypnosis. Our purpose in writing is to raise awareness and promote opportunities for giving fast paced help to professionals who work in fast paced medical procedure environments. The key term here is *fast.* This is not about the hypnosis you may have seen in the movies—the one featuring the devious villain with the mesmerizing stare or dangling watch. Our techniques also have nothing to do with lengthy sessions on a psychoanalytical couch. We know you have no time to waste.

Each chapter in *Patient Sedation Without Medication* builds on the preceding ones. We recommend that you read the entire book through in sequence, experience the Opportunities to Practice at the end of each chapter and then go back to focus on the parts you choose. The book has three parts.

Part I: Establishing Instant Rapport

Part II: Shaping the Patients' Experience

Part III: Guiding Patients in Self-Hypnotic Relaxation

For Part III in particular, you should have knowledge of all the chapters in the entire Part before deciding to apply the individual techniques.

Although *Patient Sedation Without Medication* gives adequate information to help you implement these thoroughly tested rapport and procedure hypnosis techniques, we do encourage you to further and broaden your knowledge and experience. For additional information and on-site training opportunities with Hypnalgesics, LLC, contact Elvira Lang at **EVL@hypnalgesics.com** or visit **www.hypnalgesics.com**.

Elvira V. Lang, MD Eleanor Laser, PhD

Notice of Responsibility

The techniques, methods, strategies, information, and opinions presented in *Patient Sedation Without Medication* are believed to be accurate and represent the best judgment available to the authors based on their training and experience and on the data collected during the sixteen years of their research involving rigorous prospective randomized studies with >700 patients, which clearly showed that the use of rapid rapport and quick hypnotic techniques made medical procedures more comfortable and safer for patients.

We, the authors, freely share our experiences and the results of our research with healthcare professionals who may wish to personally select and incorporate any or all of the *Patient Sedation Without Medication* techniques, methods, and strategies that they feel would be prudent additions to their unique professional work environment. However, no action or inaction should be based solely on the information presented in *Patient Sedation Without Medication.*

The hypnosis techniques presented in this book are procedure hypnosis and their inclusion here is intended for the limited use of healthcare professionals helping patients help themselves cope with medical procedures. It is neither our intention nor do we in anyway encourage readers to attempt any other application nor expansion of these techniques. While we are confident that applied as intended these techniques will be effective and safe, we cannot and do not accept any responsibility for individual application, use, or misuse of the techniques, methods, strategies, information, and opinions presented in *Patient Sedation Without Medication.*

PART I

CHAPTER 1

Building Confidence

Case 1.1 Confidence Amid Chaos

As a medical student in Boston, and as part of her work with Dr. Lang, B—— received instruction in using rapid hypnotic techniques with patients. During a later part of her medical internship, B—— spent several months on a small island off the coast of South America and recounted the following experience. During her first week at the island hospital, B—— was assisting with a cesarean section. Due to medical complications, the patient, D——, could not be intubated. Consequently, because a breathing tube could not be inserted into the airway, the patient could not receive general anesthesia; what's more, it was too late for epidural anesthesia. Since the patient's condition was critical—she urgently needed a cesarean section—the medical team decided to operate without anesthesia. Medical resources on the island were very limited. All the medical team had on hand to supplant anesthesia at this point was skin-numbing lidocaine. They applied it liberally.

Carefully, the surgeon made the first cut, which—to everyone's relief—was tolerated by the patient without a stir. On the next cut, the patient started screaming, and although the operating physician worked as fast as possible, the patient could not endure the excruciating pain. By the time the uterus was opened, the patient was kicking, fighting, biting, yelling, screaming in pain, and trying to get off the surgery table. With the patient fighting so hard, it was impossible to deliver the baby. The patient was bleeding excessively out of her incision. As they each realized the serious blood loss and the danger for both the mother and baby, the surgeons yelled at the anesthesiologists to calm the patient down; the anesthesiologists, helpless, were unconstrained in their replies. Although three people were leaning over the patient trying to hold her still, the physicians were not able to proceed with the surgery. They could not deliver the baby or even stop the blood loss. The patient was screaming and fighting, the medical staff was yelling and struggling to hold the mother down, and blood was flying everywhere. With every passing minute, it became obvious to all that unless something was done soon, the life of both mother and baby would be lost.

Until that point B—— had just watched in disbelief, waiting for someone to step in and end this terrible situation. She had already thought of suggesting hypnosis, but she hesitated. B—— had no idea what the medical team thought of hypnosis or how they might react to her suggesting it in this life-threatening situation. The minutes passed. While the near chaos continued with the patient, B—— mentally reviewed her self-doubts about suggesting that she be allowed to apply the rapid hypnotic techniques she had learned in Drs. Lang and Laser's training sessions. Perhaps no one would listen to her. Would she be able to engage the patient in such an out-of-control situation? Also, B—— was well aware that if she attempted hypnosis and failed, she might lose face and credibility. However, at this point it was clear that no one else was going to step forward and end the crisis. "Hypnosis is possibly the last hope," she thought. B—— knew she had learned the hypnosis techniques well, and comforted somewhat by her private conclusion that, "It cannot possibly get any worse," B—— found the confidence to act. She stepped up to the table.

B—— told the staff in a firm voice that she might be able to help and that she just needed to talk to the patient for a couple of minutes. Everyone looked at her and to her surprise they let her pass to the head of the patient. The patient was nearly out of her mind, screaming, crying and yelling in pain and fear. B—— took a breath and began. "D——, listen, I am here to help you, we will work through this together and you will be fine. All I want you to do is listen to my voice, are you ready?" The patient looked at B—— with fearful eyes. "Take a deep breath," the patient fell silent and took in breath, "and let it all out, that's good, and another deep breath." The patient was listening carefully to B—— and following her instructions. "It's alright, you are safe now," said B——, "I will help you through this, just keep focusing on your breathing; in... and out..." The surgery room fell into silence; everyone was watching and waiting to see what would happen next. The patient was breathing evenly, her body slowly relaxed, the screaming and fighting stopped completely and her blood pressure and heart rate returned to normal again. B—— then guided the patient to go, in her mind, home to her hammock at the beach, a familiar, comfortable place. Once the patient was imagining herself at home, B—— had her focus on the waves and blue sky of this favorite place—easily and simply, nothing spectacular, just the familiar and safe.

After several minutes into the hypnosis, B—— nodded to the surgeons to continue and they very carefully moved forward to complete the surgery. Everyone else on the medical team watched quietly as the physician approached the incision to finally deliver the baby. The patient—still focusing on B——'s voice—did not move. What a relief! Working quickly, the physicians completed the surgery within 20 minutes with the patient drifting through the procedure in deep hypnosis. The surgery was successful, and both mother and baby fully recovered. The medical staff expressed their appreciation and respect for B——'s work. The next day the mother was so grateful for B——'s heroic intervention that she named her own baby girl B——. ***Case Notes, Elvira Lang***

What This Case Illustrates Knowledge and skill are necessary and important, but they alone are not enough to make a practitioner effectual. Just as important is having the confidence to act on what one knows. Knowing what to do, but being afraid to do it, benefits no one.

The Role of Confidence

Confidence is the expectation of a positive outcome. From your first case on, it is important to step up to the plate with confidence and be determined to use what you have learned about patient sedation without medication. Don't delay your first application of patient sedation without medication until a "perfect" case comes along. Step up at your first opportunity to apply your skills regardless of whether the patient is relatively calm or the situation is so critical that you feel "nothing can make this worse." Your very act of stepping forward and taking action will raise expectations for positive outcomes. These positive expectations invariably become self-fulfilling prophecies. Stepping up with confidence in one case brings on more confidence, which then nurtures confidence for the next case, and so on in a natural building progression of greater and greater confidence, leading to more and more success.

Rosabeth Moss Kanter of Harvard Business School extensively researched the effect of confidence on winning streaks of sports teams, businesses, and even nations.(1) She defined confidence as the "sweet spot between arrogance and despair," between "assuming complacent invulnerability" and "failing to acknowledge one's strength." Approaching a patient with overbearing reliance on one's title and credentials and failing to make efforts to establish rapport is as self-defeating as being so insecure that you do not act and, thus, deprive patients of help when they need it most.

Moss Kanter puts forward the idea that confidence needs a firm foundation built on three cornerstones. One cornerstone is accountability—you've learned the facts, developed the skills and know you can take responsibility and be accountable for your performance in a given situation. Another cornerstone is collaboration—you are not the sole hero, but you help others, including patients, to achieve their best. The third cornerstone of confidence is initiative—this cornerstone combines the actions you take in a specific situation with the sense that you are responsible for and in control of those actions.

Confidence is contagious. Your acting with confidence can foster confidence in others. Roland Neuman and Fritz Stack at the University of Würzburg, Germany showed in a series of experiments that listening to another person's emotional expression automatically elicits a congruent mood in the listener.[(2)]

The need for confidence also applies to the patient. It is important to nurture confidence in the patient through your own expressions of confidence; including your posture, demeanor, and tone of voice along with what you say. Remember, a patient may have never experienced hypnosis before or may only be familiar with hypnosis in the context of stage performance or a mystery-shrouded movie. Take time to help the patient develop realistic expectations about the process he or she is about to experience.

Finally, confidence gives rise to more confidence in a medical team. Healthcare professionals armed with knowledge of the strong clinical research basis of *Patient Sedation Without Medication* and skilled in the techniques will be able to implement those techniques with confidence. When they do, their team members will have confidence in the professional, as well as in the use of hypnosis.

Expectations

Confidence in the techniques presented in *Patient Sedation Without Medication* begins with knowledge. After having conducted one pilot and three large prospective randomized studies with >700 patients, we have documented overwhelming evidence that the methods of this book work in the procedure room.[3-5] Moreover, the randomized studies also showed how much less well patients fare who do not have hypnosis. *Patient Sedation Without Medication* does not imply that all patients subjected to these techniques will enter a deep trance, and experience zero pain or anxiety. Drugs cannot make this guarantee either. However, one point is clear; patients will do ultimately better with hypnotic techniques than without them. Patients should definitely have the option of hypnosis available.

Applying the Skills and Knowledge You Have Achieved

Learning and practicing new skills is rewarding and often fun, but it does take a bit of courage. The Script that follows is an opportunity for you to experience self-hypnosis and a sense of confidence and inner strength. Make yourself comfortable. You might uncross your legs and adjust your body position until you are at ease. Now, slowly read the following script aloud or silently, as you wish. Alternatively, you could record the script on a tape and play it back—but make sure you do not listen to the tape while driving or performing attention-demanding activity.

Script 1.1 Experiencing Confidence

Take a few slow breaths in and out. You may want to say to yourself with each breath in "strength;" and with each exhale imagine you blow out tension as you breathe out. You might notice how with each inhalation you take in more strength and confidence and with exhalation you let go of even more tension. You may want to do this a few times at your own rhythm, naturally and comfortably. And as you take a few moments to enjoy these liberating breaths, notice how breathing in this way makes you feel.

Now, you can float to a time when everything just worked out well for you, one of those "magical" moments when everything just "clicked" and came together for you. It may have been a private moment or a public achievement, when something came true and through for you because you worked hard. You might have persevered and succeeded, or something just happened, something good, something good just by itself. Or when something you had learned came in very handy—one of these moments when you realize that you know how to meet the needs of the situation. And you say, "Yes! This is it!" and you fully experience the delight of this feeling. If you cannot think of such a personal experience like that right now, imagine what it might be like to have such an experience. Perhaps you have seen an experience like that in a movie, or have heard a story about someone having such an experience. Put yourself fully into that scenario.

Good. Now float further down into this magical moment in which everything just works out well. Enjoy this moment and savor the sights and sounds; wrap the feelings of achievement and delight around you.

You might even notice a color that permeates the scene. If so, you can make this "your color" and whenever—later in your work and life—you wish to regain this wonderful state of accomplishment, confidence, and peace, you may just want to think of this color. You may even want to keep at hand an object of "your" color to remind you how to enter that state of self-assurance whenever you need it, but just thinking of the color can be a signal in itself. Or there may be a sound or song in the air that can be your reminder of this moment, and just recalling this sound or song can transport you back to this state of strength whenever you wish or need to.

Alternatively, you can put thumb and forefinger together while immersed in the experience, and, hereafter, you can use this touching of the thumb and forefinger as a signal to bring to you this feeling of accomplishment, confidence, and peace that you are enjoying now. You can use one or more of these techniques whenever you desire or need to return to that confident state, even in the toughest of circumstances.

One more thing, your unconscious mind has been going through a process of allowing itself to assimilate and organize all the information that you needed into a format that your conscious mind could easily use at any time. Although you may not be fully conscious of what your unconscious mind has processed, bring that information with you as you slowly float back above yourself.

When you are ready to return to your natural state of awareness, slowly count backwards from three to one, as follows: On three, take a deep breath in. On two, let a breath out. On one, be fully awake, delighted, and proud to know how you can use your mind to relax, and how you can use your mind to help yourself and to help others. ***End of Script 1.1***

In the upcoming chapters, you will learn new skills and improve the ones you already have. You can have high expectations for success—all techniques presented in this book have been rigorously tested in practice to ensure they produce the desired results. Approaching the patient with these facts in mind will help you to create a climate of confidence that nurtures success. Patients will feel your confidence and become confident themselves. *Patient Sedation Without Medication* is about leading by example and helping patients to help themselves.

Key Points to Remember

- Knowing what to do, but being afraid to do it, benefits no one.
- Positive expectations become self-fulfilling prophecies.
- Confidence is contagious. Your acting with confidence can foster confidence in others.
- It is important to nurture confidence in the patient through your own demonstration of confidence including your posture, demeanor, and tone of voice, along with what you say.
- *Patient Sedation Without Medication* does not imply that all patients subjected to these techniques will enter a deep trance and experience zero pain or anxiety. However, one point is clear; patients will do ultimately better with hypnotic techniques than without them.
- Once you are skilled in the techniques and understand the strong clinical research base of *Patient Sedation Without Medication,* you will be able to successfully implement hypnosis techniques with confidence.

Opportunities to Practice

Next time you need to exchange an item at the store, want the sales clerk to assist you, enter a patient room to draw blood, or do a task you ordinarily do with other people: approach with confidence. Experiment with the techniques presented in script 1.1, "Experiencing Confidence": breathing in strength and blowing-out tension; going into "your color"; imagining hearing "your sound or song," or touching your thumb and forefinger to bring your body back to remembering how it feels to be confident and successful. Notice which of the approaches work best for you—alone or in combination. Notice the reaction in yourself and in the person with whom you are interacting. Do you notice a greater willingness to go along with your suggestions? Do you fulfill your tasks with greater ease and more efficiency?

CHAPTER 2

Balancing Closeness and Distance

Case 2.1 Space Issues

The newly hired member of the hospital procedure team seemed self-assured and congenial enough until it was time for Board Rounds. During this daily morning event, about 10 members of the procedure team would crowd in front of a wallboard on which the day's cases were listed. As the team gathered to discuss the cases, the new team member C—— appeared tense and kept stepping backwards, away from the group. During the next few weeks, it became clear to Dr. Lang that this person had strict space boundaries. When anyone came closer than 4 feet, C—— became observably tense. If someone came closer than 3 feet, C—— started to take backward steps, even when doing so resulted in moving to a precarious position. In one instance, C—— stepped backward into a small opening between a computer desk and a wall, and from this jammed, but apparently more comfortably-distanced spot, tried to continue the conversation. This moving-away behavior repeated itself regularly. C—— likely was not consciously aware of this personal behavior and the rest of the team did not appear compelled to make extra space for C——. The same dynamics unfolded when C—— met one-on-one with patients or co-workers. Sometimes, when C—— would step back, the conversation partner would step forward. C—— would take another step back; the partner would take another step forward until there was no more room to escape. Unfortunately, communication goals were undermined and sometimes totally derailed by C——'s need for space—particularly when a conversation partner would not or could not accommodate that need.

Whenever she encountered C——, Dr. Lang took great care in respecting this person's need for space by keeping at least 4 feet between herself and C——. This accommodation to C——'s needs required Dr. Lang to adjusted her own space preference, which is a somewhat shorter distance. After working together a few years and as mutual trust and acceptance developed, Dr. Lang was able to have a good conversation with C—— at about 3 feet apart without C—— backing up or becoming noticeably tense. However, Dr. Lang also always took the precaution of not starting a conversation where there was not enough room for one of them to step back to allow for additional distance if needed. ***Case Notes, E. Lang***

What This Case Illustrates People vary in their preference for personal space—the distance that an individual strives to maintain between himself or herself and other people during social interaction. Some people want to stand quite close during any interaction; some others prefer keeping a considerable distance. Many people can adapt subconsciously to a mutually agreeable space arrangement during an interaction. Some individuals, however, are rigidly dependent on their preference—particularly in a stressful situation. When the space needs of these rigidly-dependent individuals are thwarted, interaction is impaired. Rapport is impeded and the odds of reaching understanding are diminished.

Affecting Boundary Needs

In explaining personal space preferences, hardwiring is one factor to consider. Humans begin their lives with a need for very close contact. Brain and body chemistry promote closeness between infants and their mothers as a way to provide nutrition and warmth to the child, and to keep threats at bay.[1] At the same time, humans are hardwired to equate distance from strangers and the unknown with safety. When threats are at a safe distance, the forebrain is activated to maximize the ability to critically assess options and solutions. However, once a threat closes in, the midbrain becomes more active, and without more complex forebrain thinking, triggers the fight or flight responses in an effort to restore distance.[2] Yet, some people may need more closeness to feel safe, particularly in a threatening situation where they need the feeling of being protected and understood—just as they had been, as infants in their mother's arms.

How the competing impulses between closeness and distance play out in a person's further development and adult perception is highly individual. For most people the personal space boundary needs are somewhat flexible and sensitive to environmental factors. For example, the less light there is, the greater is the need for distance.[3] A 1980 study on personal space preferences of hospitalized adults concluded that preferred distances for hospitalized adults were less than the preferred distances at home.[4] There is also evidence that kinship or perceived relationship affects boundary needs. In the above 1980 study when patients were asked to place representations of others in proximity to their "self" silhouette, patients placed family members closest, followed with increasing distance for a doctor, a nurse, and, furthest away, a stranger.

Personal sense for space is a powerful factor to consider when building rapport. Fortunately, research is ongoing. One recent example is that of Lawrence E. Williams and John A. Bargh who, in a series of experiments at Yale University, have found evidence that a person's feelings of distance can temper the emotional intensity of stimuli.[5] Additionally, they found that feelings of emotional distance can be triggered by physical cues in the environment without reference to the self. In other words, spatial relations of objects within that environment by themselves can affect people's judgment and shape their experience.

Accommodating Personal Space Needs of Patients

When you converse, are you an "in your face" talker or do you stay at arm's length? Do you need breathing room or prefer shoulder-to-shoulder closeness during interactions? Spatial needs and preferences vary from person to person. Keeping a balance between closeness and distance with the patient (or any other communication partner) critically determines how the interaction unfolds. Although most people find equilibrium and adjust to mutually acceptable distances during a conversation, some individuals, as seen in case 2.1, "Space Issues," are strongly anchored in their preference and cannot easily adapt. Discomfort with closeness can be a professional impediment. In the case of our colleague in the "Space Issues," case," inability to cope with closeness interfered with professional effectiveness, and sometimes put people off.

Whatever a person's usual ability to automatically adapt to another's personal space needs, that ability is likely to be diminished under stress. During medical encounters, patients typically feel stressed and may have less sense for the subconscious registration and adaptation of the healthcare provider's needs for personal space. The rules of engagement should be that the patient determines the mode of interaction and the healthcare worker adjusts to facilitate instant rapport. The key is to recognize one's own needs and learn to accept and accommodate the conversation partner's needs.

Some patients want to be very close; and if the healthcare provider backs off from them, these patients can feel rejected. When a patient moves toward you, do not back away; stay where you are. Certainly, holding still may require some practice if you are not comfortable being so close. However, just holding the closeness for a moment before backing slightly away often will suffice to make the other person feel understood. On the other hand, if you notice someone backing away when talking, note the distance where the other person stops. Keep that interval as a safe communication distance whenever you interact with him or her, even if you prefer to be closer. If a person aggressively moves toward you, stand tall, remain friendly, and be firm. If you must move, step sideways but not backwards. A little observation and accommodation on your part can often evolve into a balance that feels good for both conversation partners.

Height Differences

When seeking a balance between too close and too far with a patient, you need to consider vertical spatial relationships as well as horizontal ones. Standing towering over a patient who is seated or is on a bed, procedure table, or gurney projects a power difference. Remember not to stand over people who are seated or on a gurney or are in bed. Instead, take a chair to sit next to them or bend down to be at their level. When meeting children or persons much shorter than you, bend down to be at their eye level. The following Journal Entry illustrates why adjusting height is especially important when interacting with children.

JOURNAL ENTRY 2.1

The Lady with the Black Teeth

In my initial discussion with a new patient, I soon noticed that she never smiled; not once; not ever. The reason soon came to light—black teeth. The patient was very ashamed of her teeth, which were black with decay. The woman had a severe dental phobia. The last time she had visited a dentist was when she was five years old. She was now thirty-five years old. During treatment, I was able to trace the source of the patient's anxiety about going to a dentist to that long ago dental appointment when she was five. It seems that at that appointment, the dentist's nurse had threatened the child to frighten her into keeping still during the dental procedure. The nurse warned her, "Don't you move or else the dentist will come in and pull out all your teeth." As alarming as that statement was, through guided recollection, I was able to discover that it was not the main cause of the patient's dental phobia. That five-year-old child from the past was very small. The nurse was quite tall; towering over the child in a menacing way. This recollection revealed the underlying issue that plagued the patient. The height of the nurse was the real problem, not what she said. The patient's dental phobia and resulting black teeth began primarily as a personal space issue. ***Journal Notes, E. Laser***

Barriers

Physical barriers need additional consideration when balancing closeness and distance. Having a desk or equipment between you and the patient creates a barrier—literally and figuratively. The rule of thumb is to avoid barriers when possible and limit time behind them when they are necessary. When sitting, do not have a table or equipment between you and the patient. If equipment must be between you and the patient during treatment, spend a moment or two with the patient away from the barrier before treatment begins. When both you and the patient are seated, choose a 45-degree angle—sitting right across a person can result in an uncomfortable staring situation. Sitting side by side does not give enough opportunity for observation and carries connotations of a more romantic side-by-side. Sitting behind a patient may come up in psychoanalysis but has no place in the medical encounters described in this book.

Key Points to Remember

- Personal sense for space is a powerful factor to consider when building rapport.
- Although most people find equilibrium and adjust to mutually acceptable distances during a conversation, some individuals are strongly anchored in their preference.
- Whatever a person's usual ability to automatically adapt to another's personal space needs, that ability is likely to be diminished under stress.
- The rules of engagement should be that the patient determines the mode of interaction and the healthcare worker adjusts to facilitate instant rapport.
- Avoid towering over patients and adapt to their level of height.
- Avoid or limit barriers.
- One of your first priorities in an interaction with a new patient is to determine a suitable balance between closeness and distance. Base your assessment on the patient's behavior in response to your testing varying distances.
- It is important to become comfortable with patients and other communication partners who choose personal space distances that do not reflect your personal preference.

Opportunities to Practice

- Next time you are in a conversation with a colleague, friend, or stranger, be sensitive to how they respond to you moving closer or further away. Do they move towards you or away? Which distance seems to feel right for your communication partner?
- If people come closer to you than you prefer, practice accepting and adapting rather than altering the distance.

CHAPTER 3

Matching Body Position for Rapport

Case 3.1 To Match or Not to Match: That is the Question

Drs. Lang and Laser were teaching specific strategies for quickly establishing rapport to members of a medical group. The doctors had introduced the concept of matching one's conversation partner's body position as an effective way to obtain instant rapport. Dr. Laser explained that people who are in rapport with one another automatically assume matching body positions. She went on to point out that although this matching is unconsciously and instinctively assumed by people in rapport, one can actually initiate rapport where it does not yet exist simply by consciously matching the other person's body positions. When Dr. Laser finished speaking, one of the nurses protested passionately, proclaiming that she would never do this because purposely mimicking body position was way too artificial. Her colleague and friend, who sat next to her, strongly affirmed that she, too, was of exactly the same opinion. They both seemed appalled by the whole premise of matching; yet both reluctantly agreed to participate in an exercise that required them to match their partner's body position during a difficult conversation. Afterward, both reported that they had sincerely tried but just couldn't do it. They continued to express doubts about the core concept: that people had an inherent tendency to match the body po-

sitions of those with whom they are in rapport. The nurses concluded that matching just wouldn't work for them. Less than 5 minutes later, the cameraman filming the teaching session quietly alerted Dr. Lang to observe the doubting nurses. There they sat in perfectly matching semi-oblique positions with their bodies slid halfway forward on their chairs; their opposing knees crossed over, and each with a hand on her cheek in an exact mirror image of the other. Dr. Lang asked them to not move and to just observe themselves and each other. Both were first startled and then had a loud laugh when they realized that they had, indeed, unconsciously assumed identical position. They, as well as the class, now had no trouble accepting that matching body position is a natural behavior—automatically occurring among people in rapport.
Case Notes, E. Lang

What This Case Illustrates People in rapport unconsciously match or imitate one another's body positions.

Intuitive Matching

The terms *matching, mimicry,* and *imitation* are used synonymously in the literature to describe the phenomena of two individuals assuming the same or similar behaviors. The term *mirroring* is also often used interchangeably with the other terms; however, some researchers and professionals reserve *mirroring* to describe assuming the same body position or motor functions in a reversed left to right way; as though the observer was copying an image in an actual mirror. In this book, unless a distinction is specified, we use these terms—*matching, mimicry, imitation,* and *mirroring* synonymously.

Imitating another's behavior can be found among animals to various degrees but this behavior can be observed in its most evolved forms among humans.(1) Modern brain-mapping techniques suggest that an observer's perception of a behavior (body position, gestures, facial expression, speech pattern, etc.) in another person and the subsequent imitating of that behavior by the observer are facilitated through a hardwired core circuitry in the brain. This circuitry interacts with appropriate other neural systems to sustain various forms of imitative behavior.[1] Babies imitate adults' facial expressions within minutes after birth.[2] This innate common coding for observed and generated actions is presumed to enable infants' understanding that others are like them and enable a sense of empathy for others of their kind.[2]

Some of the most interesting neurobiological discoveries in mimicry initiated in experiments with monkeys, "Monkey see, monkey do." In the early 1990s, neuroscientist Giuseppe di Pellegrino and colleagues in the research group of Giacomo Rizzolatti, Director of the Department of Neurosciences at Università degli Studi in Parma, Italy, investigated the neurons in the premotor cortex of monkeys.[3] Their work revealed activation patterns specific for the type of hand movements the animals executed such as grasping, holding, or tearing. One day the experimenters noted—quite by accident—that the very pattern of motor neuron activation that experimenters had identified as occurring when the monkeys performed certain hand movements was also occurring when the monkeys were action restricted but able to observe the experimenters performing the same hand motions. Their neurons basically fired in sync with the experimenter's actions. More recent work of the same research group showed that auditory stimuli can have similar effects.[4] While monkeys are good at imitating others they also seem to enjoy being imitated. Monkeys will preferentially look at a person who is matching their movements rather than look at a person who is not matching.[5]

These research findings in monkeys stimulated further research on "mirror neurons" and their role in imitation, empathy, and social interaction. Modern MRI techniques have enabled researchers to establish the presence of mirror neurons also in humans. Hardwired circuits for imitation can be found in several areas of the human brain: circuitry in the dorsolateral prefrontal cortex, which likely facilitates imitative learning; interaction with the limbic system, which is reasoned to affect social mirroring and the ability to empathize; and simulations of facial expressions, which may transmit acknowledgment of the emotions of other people.[1]

Matching and Mismatching

Imitating actions are a way of communicating the message: "I'm like you." One advantage of being "alike" is social. People appreciate others who are like them. Imitating of others has been shown to increase acceptance and to foster harmonious social interactions.[6] So, it is not surprising that cultures or individuals who are more focused on interdependency have an even greater tendency to match the behaviors of others than do cultures or individuals who have a more independent streak either by nature or by situational variables.[7]

While matching other people's behaviors is automatic under normal conditions, we have often observed this mechanism to be inhibited when conversations are controversial or one conversation partner is in distress. This inhibition may relate back to the known tendency of humans to reduce the natural inclination to match when he or she is more concerned about self than about the interdependence between self and others.[7]

In our teaching, we often have the trainees play out an emotionally loaded conversation permitting one person to be as unreasonable and obstructive as possible. The common result is that the partners assume mismatching body positions. Part 2 of this exercise asks the agonist to match the antagonist's body language and gestures. Invariably, the interactions become much more harmonious regardless of how hard the antagonist tries to remain uncooperative. Empirical evidence, time after time, shows that matching one's conversation partner's body positions and gestures promotes harmony and facilitates rapport.

People in rapport intuitively assume matching body positions. When we see other people, we often seem to sense who is in rapport and who is not. You may have caught yourself making such assessments when watching couples in a restaurant. Have you been subconsciously observing and assessing body positions?

JOURNAL ENTRY 3.1

Matching Matters

To illustrate the effects of matching and mismatching, we asked two of our colleagues to help us film two videos in which they act out a difficult interaction. We secretly instructed Dr. G——, taking the part of the doctor, to NOT match the body position of his colleague, Dr. H——, who was to act as the patient. Dr. H—— was unaware of our directive to Dr. G——. The scenario entailed that the patient had waited some time for his procedure, and just when being brought into the procedure room, he is told by Dr. G—— that there was an emergency case and the patient (Dr. H——) would need to postpone his procedure and he must leave the room. The patient (Dr. H——) had been instructed to be as difficult as possible. He was so effective that he finally got the doctor (Dr. G——) to walk out of the room in genuine exasperation. When we showed this video clip during a panel on communication training during a national medical meeting, we explained that we had asked Dr. G—— to NOT display one specific behavior that had affected the tone of this interaction, and we challenged the audience to figure out which behavior it was. The viewers agreed that the communication went very badly but couldn't really put their finger on why. They started to describe behaviors or omissions of which Dr. G—— clearly was not guilty. Assessments ranged from his not having introduced himself and his not having explained what was happening, to his not listening to the patient. Fortunately there was a replay button on the video, and more than one viewer had to admit to having overlooked the introduction, the initial handshake, the explanation, and the listening. Next we showed a second video with the same actors. In this second video, Dr. G—— again played the doctor and again received secret instructions. This time he was asked to match all body movements of the patient. Despite his best efforts to be obnoxious, the patient (Dr. H——) just could not stay aggressive and unreasonable. Also, Dr. G—— did not feel the genuine stress he had experienced during and after the non-matching interaction in the first video. The audience rated Dr. G——'s behavior highly in this second video; but they could not figure out what the one behavior was that Dr. G—— had displayed during the second video and avoided during the first one. When we replayed the second scenario, we did get some great laughs about the matching which now was quite obvious. ***Journal Notes, E. Lang***

How to Match

Matching does come with an important caveat. When matching, it is important to avoid the sort of mimicking that could evoke ridicule. There are two safeguards against such a connotation. First, you can safeguard against having a conversation partner perceive your actions as mocking, by slightly delaying your mirroring action. Wait just for a brief moment or so before matching. The second safeguard is to avoid continuous 100% mirroring playback. Instead, match with opposites. For example, if the partner adjusts his or her glasses by using the thumb of his or her right hand to lift the center of the frame into place, you might adjust yours—after a delay—with the thumb of your left hand. Matching is effective whether a position is mirrored exactly—such as when both communication partners cross their arms, or mirrored symbolically, such as when the observed partner crosses arms, and the observer crosses hands; or when the observed partner crosses legs at thigh level, and the observer crosses at ankle level; or when the observed partner touches his or her right ear, and the observer touches his or her left ear.

Matching to establish rapport is not limited to mirroring body position. It is also helpful to match communication cues, for example, if you observe that your conversation partner is looking down and away, you can match that action as well. Another factor to consider is rhythm of speech. If the person speaks slowly with frequent pauses—perhaps to check for comprehension cues from you—mirror that pace. If the person's speech pattern is breezy and quick, avoid giving long pedantic explanations.

Matching patients' behavior may occasionally violate what is considered "proper" demeanor of a healthcare professional. Sitting straight up with an open body position towards the patient or conversation partner often is touted as the professional posture. However, even researchers who once supported this upright, open posture as the desirable and most effective approach based on agreeable-setting experiments, had their beliefs dispelled when they evaluated subjects engaged in confrontational conversations. Under such confrontational circumstances, both conversation participants leaning away from each other resulted in greater rapport than did the usual interchange of one person (the professional) attempting to lean forward regardless of what the other person did.[8]

Key Points to Remember

- Imitating others is hardwired in the brain and an automatic natural occurrence.

- People in rapport tend to match one another's body position.
- When people are stressed or self-focused, they tend to match less.
- Active matching rapidly produces a sense of rapport and emotional understanding.
- When matching, just slightly delaying your matching action and avoiding continuous 100% playback will help avoid the sort of mimicking that could evoke ridicule.

Opportunities to Practice

- Dig out a group photo and observe who is in rapport. Do people standing next to each other assume similar positions; does matching jump from one row to the next? Where do people hold their hands or how do they turn their bodies? You may be amused to find who matches whom. If you have annual photos of the same working group, it may be interesting to notice how some people who matched before, do not do so any longer or vice versa. If you know the politics of the place, this becomes even more interesting.
- Observe the body positions of people around you and your own and use matching as an indicator of who is in rapport. Particularly if several of you have read this chapter or been trained in matching—you may spontaneously find yourself in a "Rapport Fest" (as we sometimes call it laughingly when we suddenly find all of us in identical mirror images during a meeting).

CHAPTER 4
Matching Rhythm to Lead

Case 4.1 Screaming in the Hallway

The patient's wife had just been informed that his condition was serious and that another procedure would need to be performed on him the next day. The couple, who had been married for over 50 years, had just moved to the United States. During their life together, they had experienced tremendous hardship; and through it all, the husband had always taken care of his wife and been her emotional support. Facing the possibility of losing the man who meant so much to her was unbearable for the woman; she became increasingly upset. She ran into the hallway and started to scream, gesticulate, and insult the hospital staff and employees. She just couldn't stop herself. The team was ready to call security. Dr. Lang asked them to hold off a minute, approached the screaming woman and began interacting with her by matching her actions. Dr. Lang matched the woman's wild gesticulations and loud voice as much as possible. Dr. Lang swung her arms up and down as vigorously as the woman did, and answered the screamed questions and laments in nearly as loud a voice as the woman's. After about a minute, Dr. Lang gradually shortened the excursions and speed of her arm movements, took deeper and slower breaths, and gradually lowered her voice. The patient followed Dr. Lang's lead and in no time they were both talking at a more subdued level until the woman was responding with some control and in a way more befitting to the seriousness of the situation.

Dr. Lang's initial voice and movements were likely very "inappropriate" for a doctor, but this nontraditional way of responding to the patient's wife was needed to establish a bond of rapport between herself and the distraught woman. Granted it may have been startling to see a doctor yell and gesture wildly even for a few moments, but doing so was definitely more helpful than standing by and having the distressed and overwhelmed woman escorted away by security. ***Case Notes, E. Lang***

What This Case Illustrates Rapport is quickly achieved by matching the rhythm of a person's body position, gestures, voice, or breathing patterns. At the beginning, the person you mirror determines the rhythm. Once you are both in sync, you can change pace and thereby lead by example towards more desirable behaviors.

Matching to Lead

The same principle you learned in chapter 3, "Matching Body Position for Rapport," applies to matching the rhythm of gestures, tonality and speed of voice, or breathing patterns. For example, if a patient speaks in a slow and depressed voice, a cheerful chatter could be perceived as lack of understanding. On the other hand, if the patient were loudly gesticulating as in case 4.1, "Screaming in the Hallway," responding in motionless calm would likely infuriate the person even further.

While matching of the patient can help you to quickly establish rapport, neither you nor the patient want to become stuck in a state of distress, sadness, or unhealthy physiology. Your ultimate goal is to bring the patient to a more resourceful state of greater emotional and physiological equilibrium. To reach that goal, make use of the fact that matching is a two-way street.[1; 2] When you stay with the patient and match his or her rhythm until you are both in sync, the patient will unconsciously start to match you, too. Your modeling of changes in rhythm will help the patient to break his or her current state and be led by your example towards a more resourceful state—a state in which the patient will feel better.

Distressed patients often breathe rapidly or in a shallow, constricted fashion. The focus of matching rhythm to lead in this context is to guide the patient to relax and to breathe deeply and regularly. This goal can be achieved quickly. Matching the breath for a few moments and then taking a deep breath, exhaling slowly with a quiet *ahh,* and assuming an open chest position can quickly re-equilibrate a patient.

If a patient is slumped over, sad, you can assume a similar position and speak in a low soft voice for a moment or two, and then lead toward a position of confidence with audible deep inhalation and peaceful exhalation. As shown in the Journal Entry below, such simple efforts may even be able to help you avoid having to intubate a patient in distress.

JOURNAL ENTRY 4.1

The Ultimatum

A man who sustained a motor vehicle accident was brought to the emergency room on a trauma board—his body and neck immobilized. His eyes, above the oxygen mask strapped to his face, were wide open and scared. His breath was very rapid. The emergency room attendant, who was very concerned that the patient would become unconscious if he were to continue this rapid superficial breathing, instructed the patient several times without success to breathe slower. Desperate, he warned the patient, "If you continue breathing like that, we will have to intubate you." Whether the patient understood or not that this meant insertion of a breathing tube, the remark didn't help to calm him down. Then one of our nurses approached the patient, introduced herself, and started to match his rapid breathing. The nurse continued at the patient's pace for a few breaths and then slowed her breath gradually to a more normal level. The patient followed, breathing more slowly. The nurse acknowledged and encouraged this change. Speaking softly she said, "Good, hmm" and continued to breathe normally and with confidence, repeating, "That's right, hmm." Matching the rhythm and leading did the job. No intubation needed. ***Journal Notes, E. Lang***

Key Points to Remember

- Match the rhythm of the patient's body position, gestures, tonality of voice, breathing pattern to establish rapid rapport.
- In rapport, there will not only be a tendency for you to match the patient but also for the patient to unconsciously match you.
- Once your and the patient's rhythm are in sync, you can lead the patient to a more resourceful state by gradually adjusting your pace toward a more beneficial position or behavior for the patient.

Opportunities to Practice

- Next time you sit around a group of people in a meeting, in the subway, in a waiting room, or restaurant, watch who is matching whom in this environment. Notice what your body position is. Are you unconsciously matching another person? If not, do so. After matching is going on for a little while, move your arm or hand or leg into a different position and notice what happens. You may be surprised that total strangers will follow your movement without seeming to be aware of it. You also might notice that you may have adjusted to another person in your surroundings.
- When you first encounter your next patient, follow his or her breathing pattern for a few breaths and then lead with a nice deep happy inhalation and exhalation. Notice what happens.

CHAPTER 5

Identifying Sensory Preferences

Case 5.1 Listening Closely

During a training session, Dr. Laser played a procedure tape in which she hypnotized a patient and guided that patient on a mental "trip" to Alaska. Throughout the tape, Dr. Laser spoke in a very matter-of-fact voice. When the tape was finished playing, I——, one of the nurse participants in the training mentioned with relief that, "After listening to Dr. Laser, it really sounds like it isn't essential to speak with what one would call a hypnotist's tone of voice." I—— said she could tell that the patient responded well to Dr. Laser's descriptions spoken in a normal tone, and was, therefore, delighted that she, too, would be able to speak normally when helping patients with self-hypnotic relaxation.

For the next group exercise in the training session, the participants were asked to practice use of imagery with one another as a means of sedation without medication. Imagery is the remembrance or imagination of a place of safety and comfort in which the patient can immerse him- or herself with all senses. I—— was teamed with a colleague who was to guide I—— on a "journey" to a vacation spot that both I—— and the colleague knew well. The colleague provided beautiful imagery; describing a walk on a winding path, told of feeling with every step the softness of the earth under her feet, and of enjoying the warmth of the sun while a soft breeze gently played with the leaves high up in the trees. The colleague was obviously charmed by her own description of this favored place. I——, however, was not nearly as enchanted. It was clear that I—— was making an effort to follow her colleague's imagery, but it was obvious that she was not relaxing. I——'s response changed quickly, however, when Dr. Laser whispered in the colleague's ear a suggestion that caused the colleague to modify her imagery accordingly. The result was success—I—— did become enchanted by the new imagery. Dr. Laser's suggestion that brought this difference on was "I—— likes auditory terms—use more of those." I—— visibly relaxed when guided by her colleague to listen to the sounds of a splashing waterfall in the distance, to hear the birds singing in the air, and to hear the gentle rustling of leaves in a mild breeze. ***Case Notes, E. Laser***

What This Case Illustrates Listening carefully to people's word choices helps identify whether their perceptual sensory preference is visual, auditory, kinesthetic, olfactory, or gustatory. Respecting their preference and including terms that reflect their preference in your own speaking helps promote rapport and structure imagery.

Perceptual Strategies

We perceive what is happening around us through the five senses: sight, sound, touch, smell, and taste. At any moment, people have a general—or situational—strategy of sensory preferences through which they experience the outer world or their inner state. Some people are relatively inflexible; they have a definite specific sensory preference or they prefer a specific sequence of sensory processing, such as first looking, then smelling, then listening.(1) Many people, conversely, are quite at ease in shifting sensory preference depending on circumstance or situation, including the companions they find themselves among. Robert Dilts and colleagues, in their book of *Neuro-Linguistic Programming (NLP)*—which serves as the standard reference text for the field—postulated a model in which information is received, organized, consolidated, and transmitted along neural pathways through internal processing strategies that each individual has learned and that affect a person's behavior and imagination.(1) These authors placed heavy emphasis on decoding a patient's sensory strategy, responding in kind, and then using that strategy to bring about desired behavior.

There has been controversy about how much "reprogramming" of a person can be achieved with NLP and about the empirical nature of the research.(2) Some concerns may have arisen out of fear of the potential for manipulative use of these techniques in non-medical settings. Modern neurophysiological methods and advanced imaging technology have brought forth evidence that brings strong credence to the concept and value of matching a conversation partner's body position, speech, etc., as explained in chapter 3, "Matching Body Position for Rapport." Thus, accepting the value of matching another person's sensory "representational" systems to enhance rapport no longer requires a leap of faith.

Matching Sensory Language

People appreciate others with whom they are "alike," or have something in common. As pointed out in chapter 3, "Matching Body Position for Rapport," you can adapt to your patient's tone of voice, facial expression, mannerisms, and gestures. One more way for the practitioner to quickly establish a commonality with a patient is to analyze the patient's language. The sensory language that a person favors reveals his or her perception strategy. Most people express themselves predominantly with words from one of the following sensory categories: visual (relating to images), auditory (relating to sounds), kinesthetic (relating to movements and feelings), olfactory (relating to smells and smelling), and gustatory (relating to tastes and tasting). For example, various patients might express a similar negative feeling about their situation in any of the following ways:

- Visual preference patient: "I don't like the looks of this."
- Auditory preference patient: "This is enough to make me scream."
- Kinesthetic preference patient: "I feel like I'm falling apart."
- Olfactory preference patient: "This stinks."
- Gustatory preference patient: "I'm getting fed up with trying to get a straight answer."

Once you determine the patient's sensory term preference, feed back what you identified by matching. Speak the patient's "language." For example, in reply to the above patients, you could say:

- To visual patient: "Are things beginning to look a little better?"
- To auditory patient: "Does that sound like something you would prefer?"
- To kinesthetic patient: "If you can hold on for just a few more seconds."
- To olfactory patient: "Have I cleared the air a little?"
- To gustatory patient: "I'll explain the procedure in small bites that are easier to digest."

In case 5.1, "Listening Closely," Dr. Laser was able to identify I——'s auditory preference by noting the sensory mode of the words that I—— used to comment in class. I—— had explained that after *listening* to Dr. Laser it really *sounds* like it isn't essential to *speak* with what one would *call* a hypnotist's *tone of voice.* She could *tell* that the patient *responded* well to Dr. Laser's *descriptions spoken* in a normal *tone,* and was therefore, delighted that she, too, would be able to *speak* normally when helping patient with self-hypnotic relaxation. The colleague who structured I——'s imagery, conversely, favored kinesthetic words, that is, her preference related to sensations, feelings, and movement. Thus, her ideal scenario was *walking* on a *winding* path, *feeling* with every *step* the *softness* of the earth *under her feet,* enjoying the *warmth* of the sun *and* a *soft* breeze while a the *wind gently played* with the leaves *high up* in the trees. I——, having a strong auditory preference, did not respond to the kinesthetically presented scenario. I—— preferred to *listen* to the sounds of a *splashing waterfall* in the distance, *to hear* the birds *singing* in the air, and to hear the gentle *rustling* of leaves. A person with a visual perceptional preference might have enjoyed envisioning the *golden* rays of the sun *reflecting* and *shimmering* on the distant waterfall in *brilliant hues of light.* A person with an olfactory preference might like to *breathe* in the *fresh* air, *smell* the *scents* of leaves, moss, and early spring flowers—the subtle *aromas* that are the *essence* of a relaxing experience. A person with a gustatory preference might *relish* the *tinge* of sunrays penetrating the canopy of leaves, *savor* the *sweet tang* of the vegetation in the wood, and enjoy the *delicious taste* of freedom a walk in the woods can bring. Reading through these examples, you may find that one speaks more to you than the others. Insight, perhaps, into your own sensory preference.

Later, when you structure imagery for hypnosis, you will want to always engage all of the senses and have the patient fully drawn into the experience through all senses. You may start with a patient's preference, but if you make a habit of always going full circle, tapping all five senses, you can't miss the preferred one, and you will be better able to provide a full immersion into the imagery process.

Words Grouped by Sensory System

To give yourself a head start, you can use the following words to help you become more conversant in describing the different sensory categories. You can expand the following list according to what you may most encounter in your surroundings:

- Visual words: *appear, bright, dark, focus, picture, envision, view, watch, pretty*
- Auditory words: *argue, call, describe, hear, listen, silent, tell, sound, quiet, ring*
- Kinethetic words: *connect, cut, grab, grasp, handle, hold, pressure, smooth, feel*
- Olfactory words: *breathe, inhale, odor, smell, stink, whiff, fragrant, stuffy*
- Gustatory words: *bite, delicious, flavor, sweet, taste, tongue, juicy, yummy*

Note that patients with olfactory and gustatory preferences tend to also be kinesthetically oriented.

Key Points to Remember

- At any moment, people have a general—or situational—strategy of sensory preferences through which they preferentially experience the outer world or their inner state.
- Some people may be quite inflexible regarding their specific sensory preference. Some other people, however, are quite at ease in shifting sensory preference depending on circumstance or situation.
- The sensory language that a person favors reveals his or her perception strategy.
- Once you determine the patient's sensory term preference, feed back what you identified by matching. Speak the patient's "language."

Opportunities to Practice

- Dictate into a microphone or write rapidly without much thinking on a piece of paper how you image your favorite vacation. Play back or read and notice which sensory terms you use preferentially.
- In your next conversation listen carefully and attempt to identify the speaker's sensory preference. Reply in kind.
- When you read an interview in a magazine identify what sensory preferences the interviewer and interviewee have and how or whether they adapt to each other during the interview.

CHAPTER 6

Interpreting Eye Position

Case 6.1 Looking Sideways

L—— and J—— both worked as nurses in the same unit for many years and shared many views on life, work, and family. Occasionally they spent time together outside of work. L——, however, always felt somewhat uneasy in J——'s presence. J——'s habit of looking to the side whenever they engaged in a conversation caused L—— to feel that J—— didn't really care about her or, at the very least, didn't value what she had to say. L—— had no reason to doubt her interpretation of J——'s lack of eye contact until she took a communication class with us. When we addressed subconscious eye movements, L—— had a profound *aha!* experience. She realized that J——'s posture and sideway gaze were simply typical expressions of an auditorily-anchored perceptual preference and not a comment on L—— or her conversation. L——'s new understanding of eye movements made her much more comfortable in J——'s presence. She no longer misinterpreted J——'s eye movements as an affront. She became more relaxed when talking with J——. What's more, L——, once she was aware of J——'s auditory preference, began to emphasize this preference in her own word choices. This change seemed to have a positive effect on J——. Their rapport deepened, and their friendship continued to develop. ***Case Notes, E. Lang***

What This Case Illustrates When engaged in conversation, people untrained in eye-movement interpretation tend to impose negative or positive messages on the eye movements of their conversation partner even though such movements are mostly involuntary and may indicate nothing more than the partner's sensory preferences.

Eye Movements and Sensory Preferences

Eye movements come into play with the sensory preferences and perceptual strategies discussed in chapter 5, "Identifying Sensory Preferences." It is within the terms of their senses—visual, auditory, kinesthetic, olfactory, and gustatory—that humans perceive the world. Although most people are able to take in the environment simultaneously with all five senses; at any given moment one or two of these senses gain perceptual priority and shape the mind's strategy for processing information. Involuntary eye movements, which may be obvious or quite subtle, accompany access to the perceptual strategy of the moment.(1)

Decoding and Interpreting Eye Movements to Establish Rapport

People's subconscious eye movements are hardwired and transcultural.(2) These involuntary eye movements are a reflection of whether an individual is mentally creating or remembering, and are an indication of his or her subconscious sensory preferences.(1) People on the receiving end often see more in these subconscious eye movements than the movements actually offer. Two factors contribute to this error. The first is simply that people are very sensitive to being looked at by others.(3) In addition, the areas in the brain that process direct and averted gaze are also involved in attributing other people's intentions and beliefs.(4) One can see how this may easily produce misunderstandings such as in case 6.1, "Looking Sideways." You can avoid such misinterpretations—and the discomfort that can accompany them—by learning to decode and interpret eye movements correctly. In addition, you can use your insight into your conversation partner's sensory focus to tailor your choice of words to support your partner's perceptual strategy as you have learned in chapter 5, "Identifying Sensory Preferences."

Sensory Preferences Indicated by Subconscious Eye Movements

Relative directions appearing below are given from your counterpart's—the observed person's—orientation. Your counterpart's *right* is your *left*. Your counterpart's *left* is your *right*. In principle, people tend to move their eyes to the left when accessing memory and to the right when constructing content. Typically, visual content is associated with upward gaze, auditory content with horizontal eye position, and kinesthetic content with downward gaze.[(1)] In essence, sensory preference indication signals may be summarized as follows:

Visual

- Eyes up and to the left: recalling imagery
- Eyes up and to the right: constructing imagery

Auditory

- Eyes same level of gaze and to the left: remembering auditory experiences
- Eyes same level and to the right: constructing sounds, putting something into words

Kinesthetic, Gustatory, and Olfactory

- Eyes down and to the right: awareness of body sensations
- Eyes down and to the left: internal dialogue; talking to oneself

Decoding and Interpreting Subconscious Eye Movements

It may come as a relief to know that the reason people don't look you straight in the eyes when you speak to them is, most of the time, not because they are dishonest or inattentive but because they are processing what you say through their own perceptional strategy. People take in the world using the perceptional strategies through which they are best able to process information. Thus, as explained above, if your conversation partner attempts to connect with personal experiences that are pertinent to what he or she hears, his or her eyes may break contact with you and shift to the left.

For persons with strong auditory sensory preferences great listening may require NOT looking at you but to look to the right or left of you. Auditorily-anchored persons may also assume a "telephone position," slightly cocking their head and holding their hand as if holding a phone to their ear.(1) Also, if the conversation involves feelings, then a downward gaze would be quite natural. A person who is kinesthetically anchored may speak slower, with more pauses. Visually processing individuals may keep looking upward and use quick bursts of words in a high pitch and have a fast tempo of speech.

There are no right or wrong sensory preferences and associated eye movements. It is important to recognize and accept that different people may have different sensory priorities in general and at a given time in any conversation. Most people can shift between sensory preferences depending on the situation. However, when stressed, most tend to adhere more rigidly to their preferred perceptual strategy.

When to Utilize Subconscious Eye Movement Awareness

You will find sensory preference awareness helpful in various settings: when you need to gauge your reaction of unease with a conversation partner; or when you want to establish instantaneous rapport with a patient and respond in a supporting way by emphasizing this preference in your own choice of words—according to the method outlined in chapter 5, "Identifying Sensory Preferences." Sensory preference awareness can be especially helpful if you find yourself in a stressful situation and may have become stuck in your preferred eye position and perceptual strategy. Being stuck in your preference is particularly problematic when it is contrary to the other person's gaze preference and expectations.

JOURNAL ENTRY 6.1

The Ups and Downs of Interviewing

The department interviewed several applicants for the position of a new secretary. P—— was highly qualified based on her professional experience and had excellent references. During the interview, she consistently looked downward and did not engage in eye contact. She spoke softly and slowly. Two of the staff rejected her on the basis of these behaviors alone. They judged her avoidance of eye contact and low-volume voice as unsuitable for the job. They said they were concerned that she would not be able to handle incoming patients, and would be too slow for the fast-paced environment. Two interviewers were lukewarm about P——, but couldn't say why. The secretarial supervisor, who was highly experienced in recruitment, and a senior faculty member, who was well aware of the traps of eye contact interpretation, decided to hire. P——, who is deeply kinesthetically anchored, performed superbly. Away from the interview stress, her eye movements were freer. She worked very efficiently and fast, was well accepted, and clearly liked by both staff and patients. ***Journal Notes, E. Lang***

Key Points to Remember

- Although most people are able to take in the environment simultaneously with all five senses; at any given moment, one or two of these senses gain perceptual priority and shape the mind's strategy for processing information.
- People's subconscious eye movements are hardwired and transcultural.
- An averted gaze does not mean that your conversation partner does not listen or has something to hide.
- A person's eye movements are a reflection of individual sensory preferences and perceptual strategies.
- Accessing memory is typically associated with a shift of the eyes to the left; constructing new content, with a shift to the right.
- Visual strategies are typically associated with upward gaze, auditory strategies with horizontal gaze, and kinesthetic strategies with downward gaze.
- Decoding and interpreting eye movements provides insight into effective ways to communicate with patients by responding to their sensory preferences.

Opportunities to Practice

- Observe and decode eye movements to interpret sensory preferences: while talking to colleagues, family members, or friends; when shopping and asking the sales person questions about a product; while watching a person being interviewed on TV.
- The next time you identify a person with a strong sensory preference, follow that preference in your word choices and note the person's reaction.
- You can check on your own sensory preference. If you can video yourself, tell a story into the camera and review later where your eyes moved and what wording you chose.

CHAPTER 7

Touching in the Medical Environment

Case 7.1 Touchy About Touching

The protocol of Dr. Lang's research studies required that the medical procedures in the trials would be videotaped to assure that the patients were actually receiving the treatment to which they had been randomized. One day, the two research assistants charged with reviewing the videotapes came, in obvious distress, to Dr. Lang's office wanting to discuss an observation. On the video that was the source of the research assistants' concern, a nurse approached a patient lying on a procedure table; stood beside the patient awhile, and then started stroking the patient's head and forehead. One of the research assistants, a psychologist, was quite concerned about this action and thought the patient had been reduced to a child-like state by the nurse's stroking. The other research assistant was concerned about propriety issues and posited that sexual innuendo could be construed. The team discussed the video and raised concerns with the charge nurse responsible for the procedure room. She was somewhat ambivalent. Undoubtedly the nurse who had stroked the patient had done so with the best of intentions and out of a sense of caring. When approached about the incident, the nurse confirmed that she was only trying to comfort the patient and was quite unaware that her actions could possibly be misinterpreted. All on the team agreed to, hereafter, obtain permission from patients before touching them, and to always exert great care when touching patients to avoid possible misinterpretations of touching actions. ***Case Notes, E. Lang***

What This Case Illustrates Because touching of a patient—regardless of the intention of the practitioner and the medical need to touch—can easily be misunderstood or be unwelcome, it is essential to ask the patient's permission before touching. It is equally important after obtaining permission to take great care about where and how you touch the patient to avoid any misinterpretation.

Liabilities in Touching

Over the years, we were surprised to find how many patients had been subjected to abusive experiences in their past. We were told of being wrapped in carpets or locked up in the dark for punishment, being raped, and being taken hostage. Unfortunately, integral to many medical procedures are powerful stimuli that can readily bring on memories of such past abuse: the patients are immobilized, possibly dressed only in a gown or nothing at all below procedure sheets, delivered to the mercy of authority, scared for their well-being, and unable to avoid physical contact. Additionally, in some procedures, such as those in radiology or gastroenterology, the lights may be turned down to better facilitate viewing of the monitors. Such a set-up can increase the risk of a practitioner's touch being misinterpreted. Patients with a history of abuse may spontaneously regress—retreat to an earlier stage of development—or dissociate—perceive a detachment of the mind from the emotional state or even from the body. These possibilities are especially likely if the practitioner's touch is perceived as sexual or similar to the behavior of a past abuser. Patients may relive the earlier experience in vivid, frightening detail (regression). Alternatively, they may attempt to separate themselves from reality (dissociation) using coping mechanisms, which, although they may have worked well at the time of the abuse, can be quite detrimental when displayed on the examination table. Consequently, with the exception of the initial handshake, you should not touch a patient without his or her clear, explicit permission. Furthermore, even with verbal permission, it is important to pay close attention to a possible nonverbal, "No." Because they may be embarrassed or feel too intimidated to refuse, patients might give permission when they would rather not. If the patient hesitates before answering or tenses up, it could be a signal that although the verbal message was "yes, go ahead," the actual message may well be "Stop! I don't want to be touched."

Touching in Social and Medical Settings

Social tactile stimulation is important for normal development. Beyond the early needs of children for closeness and its corollary touch—as described in chapter 2, "Balancing Closeness and Distance"—touching continues to affect human interactions. In a social context, a quick touch on the arm may have a beneficial effect for the "toucher." Nicolas Guéguen showed in several studies that touching a person's arm for a second results in a more positive evaluation of the toucher by the person who was touched. The touch also increases compliance by the touched person with a request made by the toucher—such as following suggestions of a waitperson, leaving a bigger tip, being more positive towards a car salesman, or being more willing to help strangers on the street.[1; 2] Vincent Drescher and coworkers, in an experimental series involving healthy consenting volunteers, showed that touching another person on his or her wrist for 30 seconds reliably reduces heart rate in a reflex-like fashion.[3] Note that in all of the above touching examples, the touch actions were fleeting in nature, targeted towards the distal extremities, and without suspicion of covert sexual or superiority connotations.

There may be some medical benefit in touching. In the coronary intensive care unit, James Lynch and colleagues found that palpating the pulse resulted in a reduction of high-frequency extraventricular beats in the minute immediately after pulse palpation. In these cases, the action involved touching the distal extremity in ways not typically associated with romantic or sexual aspirations, and expected as part of performance of a professional duty. However, practitioners must take care to not be perceived as forcing their authority even in cases where there is no doubt about permission to touch or there is actually an invitation from the patient to do so. For example, even in the act of holding hands, hierarchies develop depending on whose hand is in the uppermost—controlling—position.(4) Typically when men and women hold hands, the man's hand is in the uppermost position. When an adult holds hands with a child, the adult's hand is usually on top of the child's hand. You may remember this when a patient asks for his or her hand to be held during a procedure. You can comply with the request, but remember to have the patient hold onto to you in such a fashion that you do not imply superiority.

In the clinical context, expectations and acceptability standards may change from those applied during social encounters. Carole Esterbrooks and Janice Morse suggest that "Nurses have the permission of society to violate norms, and touching others intimately is a component in the routine accomplishment of many nursing tasks."(5) The same authors also acknowledge that teaching touching is one of the most neglected areas in nursing education. They report that norms of how nurses touch patients develop from three major factors: whether the nurses come from "touchy" families or not, what they observe in the behavior of more senior nurses, and in how the patient reacts to initial touching. It is the habit of many nurses to assume permission if there is no explicit patient response to the contrary. Rather than assuming a "yes" we favor asking for permission. A simple "Is it ok to touch? " will do. It does not take extra time before a pulse check to ask, "May I take your pulse?" It is also important not to be offended if the patient indicates verbally or nonverbally that touching is not desired, and to suppress any desire that might arise for mutuality in touching.

When touching the "where" and "how" of the action become important factors. Medical needs determine the area of physical contact in many cases. When there is a choice, as for giving comfort to a patient on a procedure table, the shoulder offers a good location to touch. The shoulder is typically not associated with abusive or sexual connotations. Since patients may come with preexisting pains, it is important to avoid potentially painful regions unless necessary at the stage of diagnostic evaluation. You may use a flat hand or a rounded grasp depending on the patient's preference or reaction. When using a pointed finger the pressure should be light enough so that no skin indentations result.

Touching as a Means of Anchoring

Although there may be potential pitfalls in deciding to touch a patient, touching can have positive effects. Appropriately done in the right setting and with permission, touch can be a powerful tool. One highly effect use of touch in hypnosis is anchoring. Just as a maritime anchor locks a ship in a specific location, hypnotic anchoring locks in the subject's connection to a specific experience and its attending feelings.[6; 7] You may recall in script 1.1, "Experiencing Confidence," when you experienced a great moment of confidence, self-fulfillment, and calm. We suggested that you associate with that experience a color, a sound, or the touching of your thumb with your forefinger and explained that you could use this signal whenever you needed to bring yourself back into this wonderful state at a moment's notice. Depending on the person's preference or situation, an anchor can be visual, auditory, or kinesthetic. The following journal entry illustrates using touch as an anchor with a patient.

JOURNAL ENTRY 7.1

Going With the Flow

A man came in for an interventional procedure. He was very anxious. In preparation for his procedure, I began a conversation with him, hoping to gain insight into what would be an appropriate and appealing context for him to experience in hypnosis. I asked what he did to make a living. He replied boating and touring. I inquired further how he feels when he's on the water. He said water is not only his work, but his passion. With that information, I looked no further—we headed out to sea.

As I described floooooating on the boat on a calm, clear day, the water was still and as we threw a pebble down into the water, we watched as it began to descend. As I was describing the floating and the deepening of the pebble in the water, the patient began to blink. At that blink, I anchored him to the experience by placing my hand on his right shoulder. I held my hand there, and as I described the pebble floating down further and deeper on this beautiful day; he began to slump and relax his face and entire body. As the pebble floated down even further in the water, he became even more relaxed, and I put my hand again on his shoulder to anchor this present feeling. I told the patient, "From now on, you can always feel this calm sense of floating and peace from your memory, and your memory alone. You can enjoy this relaxation that you are experiencing now at anytime you choose, even during the height of your procedural experience. When you want to return to this safe, pleasant time, just imagine a hand on your shoulder and go with the flow. ***Journal Notes, E. Laser***

Purposely anchoring a person is a very helpful technique. The key point to consider here is how easily anchoring can occur. Although in journal entry 7.1, "Going With the Flow," Dr. Laser included a formal explanation and suggestion to the patient with the anchor of her hand touching the shoulder; in our experience, an explanation is not always necessary. Just placing a hand on the shoulder when the patient is experiencing a resourceful state can anchor such positive feelings. Because a simple touch can anchor the feelings the patient is experiencing at that moment, you want to consider the patient's state before you touch. Be mindful that patients visiting a hospital or medical office are already in a highly suggestible state and you would not want your touch to anchor a patient to feelings of fear, pain, and distress. The possibility of inadvertent anchoring is another good reason to be careful of when and where and how you touch.

Key Points to Remember

- Always ask for permission to touch before you touch.
- Touching, even when well intended and medically necessary, can be misinterpreted to have sexual connotations or imply a superiority/inferiority relationship.
- Even when there is no doubt about permission to touch, care must be taken so as not to be perceived as forcing one's authority.
- When touching, make sure the area chosen is not painful due to an underlying medical condition.
- When touching with a finger, be sure that the pressure does not leave indentations.
- Because touch can anchor the feelings the patient is experiencing at that moment, you must be careful to consider the patient's state before you use an anchoring touch on him or her.

- The shoulder is often a good location for touch and also for anchoring in supine patients since it typically does not have sexual connotations.

Opportunities to Practice

Observe when your colleagues touch a patient and how the patient reacts. Do your colleagues ask for permission? Do you think the patient has a choice in being touched? What do you think are reasons for the touching—medically needed, for the sake of the patient, or for the sake of the healthcare provider?

PART II

CHAPTER 8

Avoiding Negative Suggestions

Case 8.1 Ready to Sting and Burn?

Large core breast biopsy involves inserting a large hollow needle through the skin to the site of the abnormal growth to collect and remove a sample of cells for analysis. Typically, the procedure begins by numbing first the skin and then an underlying tissue tract towards the suspicious area. Local anesthetic is administered through a thin needle. The patient is conscious during the entire procedure. Following are verbatim excerpts from 20 minutes of a recorded conversation during the first step of an actual large core breast biopsy procedure—the injection of local anesthetic through the skinny needle.

[The patient is prepped and draped. The doctor is ready to give the local anesthetic.]

Doctor: Okay, you are going to feel a pinch, and a lot of burning and stinging.

[The doctor starts giving the anesthetic.]

Doctor: This is a pinch....A pinch....okay.

Doctor: Burning and stinging. How are you doing? Doing okay?

Doctor: Pinch and sting.

[The doctor gives more local anesthetic.]

Doctor: Do you feel that? More stinging.
Patient: I can still feel a needle in there.
Doctor: You feel a needle, but do you feel any sharp pain?
Patient: I am okay. I just feel a needle.
Doctor: You feel a something moving but nothing painful, nothing sharp, right?
Patient: Uh...I feel prickly...yeah.
Doctor: What was that? Sharp?...Sorry.
Patient: That hurts!
Doctor: Sorry.
[The doctor removes the needle and her hand.]
Patient: That kills. It hurts ... it hurts! It hurts!
Doctor: There is nothing there.
[The doctor places a gauze on the puncture site.]
Doctor: Does it still sting?
Patient: It didn't sting before...weren't you doing it before?
Doctor: I will give you some more local.
Patient: Wait, wait, wait. What did you just do? The last three times you injected me didn't hurt. It stung a little. But this time it feels like you are cutting the flesh out of my chest.
Doctor: Sorry about that.
Doctor: Is it burning now?
Patient: (No response)
Case Notes, E. Lang

What This Case Illustrates The all too common practice of using negative words such as *pinch, burn,* and *sting* to "warn" patients that the about-to-be-felt sensations from procedure stimuli are going to be painful or unpleasant can become a self-fulfilling prophecy.

The Power of Negative Suggestions

Concerns about not knowing their diagnosis and about possible serious effects of treatment can be great stressors and sources of anxiety for patients seeking medical intervention.[1; 2] Patients in this situation are vulnerable to a pessimistic interpretation of information they are soaking up.[3] Words, tone, expressions, and context determine if the information received creates positive or negative expectations.[4] Negative expectations bring about negative outcomes.[5] Bayer and colleagues showed in experiments with sham stimulations that volunteers who expected pain reported pain, even when there were no painful stimuli.[4] It follows that when healthcare providers make distressing predictions about the sensations patients are about to experience, as documented in case 8.1, "Ready to Sting and Burn?" those predictions can create new specific fears previously beyond the patient's imagination.

Qualifiers Don't Mitigate

Negative suggestions, such as those discussed above, have an effect even when they are preceded by a *no, not,* or *little.* The mind takes on the image and disregards the qualifiers. Our research showed that such negative suggestions as compared to none at all or to neutral ones, when used as warning of upcoming stimuli, increase pain perception and anxiety.[6] Also, when used to sympathize after a painful stimulus, negative suggestions have been found to increase patients' anxiety. The easiest way to give your patients a better experience is to simply avoid such statements.

When Don't Means Do

Try this experiment: For the next three minutes, do not think of bananas. Don't picture *bananas;* don't say bananas in your mind; don't recall banana experiences. How did you do? There is a good chance that before you read the experiment, you were not thinking about bananas. There is an even better chance that once you did read the experiment, it became difficult for you to not think of them. The mention of the name of the fruit has raised the concept of bananas into your consciousness and now they are hard to ignore. In the medical procedure context, the same principle applies to both suggesting painful sensations and to mentioning actions that interfere with procedure progress; such as "Don't swallow," "Don't move," "Don't scratch," Don't blink," "Don't cough," or "Don't talk." Although the issuing of such suggestions and commands is well intended, the result all too often is that the concept of the desire to swallow or move or blink, etc. is suddenly raised in the patient's consciousness and once raised, is—like the bananas—difficult to ignore. Instead of issuing such commands, consider the alternatives discussed later in this chapter.

Why People Use Negative Suggestions

There seem to be two main reasons behind the use of negative suggestions in the healthcare environment. Healthcare providers who use negative suggestions either truly believe such suggestions are helpful to patients, and/or are simply repeating the vocabulary and approach they have been taught and with which they have become familiar.

At an earlier occasion, before we recorded the interaction in the "Ready to Sting and Burn?" case, we had an opportunity to talk extensively with the attending physician in that case. During this earlier conversation, we had asked the doctor about avoiding negative suggestions during procedures in keeping with a study we were performing.(7) The doctor, however, was firmly convinced that the negative-suggestion approach was not only right, but compassionate as well. Hence the doctor's surprise when the patient in the "Ready to Sting and Burn?" case finally got the message that this was supposed to hurt and said, "That kills. It hurts... it hurts! It hurts!"

Leaving the doctor to imply that the patient was imagining the pain by protesting, "There is nothing there."

JOURNAL ENTRY: 8.1

The Nurse Who Wanted to be Liked

When asked about her routine use of negative suggestions with patients during a specific procedure, a nurse defended her actions with the following explanation: She said she was well aware that the procedure was not very painful at all, but "knew" that if she were to describe it upfront as quite uncomfortable and challenging, then patients would—in the end—be very pleased and impressed with the great care they received from her to mitigate that expected pain. They would be, she theorized, very relieved that the procedure turned out to be not nearly as bad as they imagined. As shown in the "Ready to Sting and Burn?" case and other cases, this is, unfortunately, not how the mind works. ***Journal Notes, E. Lang.***

The insidious feature of using negative suggestions in the healthcare environment and the factor that helps keep them so ubiquitous in medical facilities is that the people using them keep having their assumptions proved correct. When practitioners make negative suggestions to patients about what is about to happen or is happening, the patient will, eventually, experience the suggested feelings and verbally or nonverbally express distress. The practitioner interprets these messages of distress from the patient as a clear validation of the practitioner's assumptions—"I was right, it did hurt." With this reinforcement, the practitioner might approach the next case by issuing even stronger warnings to the patient. In response, that patient might be even more distressed.

How to Avoid Negative Suggestions and Use Alternatives

Avoiding negative suggestions becomes much easier when you learn alternative approaches. Which of the following would fit into your practice?

To Prepare the Patient Before Upcoming Stimuli:

- Be descriptive and leave the interpretation up to the patient. *"I will give you the local anesthetic now."*
- Mention a competing sensation. *"I will give you the numbing medicine now. You may feel some cooling or tingling, and you may feel a sensation of warmth when the contrast medium is given."*
- Don't mention the stimulus when it is obvious what is happening. *"Can you please relax your arm over this chair?"*(while wiping off the site for a flu shot.)
- Use a neutral descriptor instead of "clinical" jargon. In MRI you may hand the patient the *"call button"* instead of *"panic button."*

To Express Empathy and to Monitor the Patient's Experience:

- Avoid "How are you?" Patients in America are socially primed to say "Okay" or "Great!" and are unlikely to give you the information you seek.
- Respect patients' right to their own experience when checking in. You may use neutral terms such as "What were (are) you experiencing?" "What are you noticing?"
- If you wish to include a kinesthetic element you can ask "How are you feeling right now?" or "What does this feel like?" If the patient has other strong sensory preferences, (See chapter 6, "Interpreting Eye Position"), you might preface your question with short statements such as "Let me see ..." or "Please

tell me how that was," or "Please describe what you are experiencing."

- Avoid "Sorry" unless you made a mistake. Instead, ask a question. "Is there anything I can do to make you feel more comfortable?"

To Encourage the Patient to Avoid Moving:

- Avoid statements that attract attention to the undesirable activity such as "Don't swallow" or "Don't move."
- If patients are not moving, it is likely they will not start to do so unless startled. No instruction is necessary in this case.
- If patients move around or you want to detract their attention, you might offer patients permission to move alternative body parts instead of the part you need to stay still. For example, you could suggest rubbing the finger tips against each other when the legs are involved in the procedure or ask the patient to focus on doing minuscule toe curls when the procedure requires working on his or her neck or arms.

To Promote a Negative-Suggestion-Free Work Environment:

- Encourage your coworkers to avoid negative suggestions by pointing to research showing their adverse effects.[4-6]
- Make and display small posters in your work area promoting the use of specific alternative non-negative vocabulary relevant to your area.
- Don't despair and don't get angry. It may take a long time to change the habits of others regarding the use of negative suggestions but eventually people will come around and learn to cherish working in a negative-suggestion-free zone.

Key Points to Remember

- Patients tend to take the practitioner at his or her word, and are likely to "feel" what they have been told they will feel.
- Negative suggestions have an effect even when they are preceded by a *no, not,* or *little.* The mind takes on the image and disregards the qualifiers.
- Suggesting painful sensations or mentioning actions that interfere with progress, such as "Don't swallow" and "Don't move," will bring these elements into the patient's consciousness; and once raised, they are difficult for the patient to ignore.
- Avoiding negative suggestions becomes much easier once you learn effective alternative vocabulary and experience the success of doing without negative suggestions.

Opportunities to Practice

- Listen to your co-workers when they talk to patients; note if they use negative suggestions. Observe the effect on the patients.
- Mentally review or speak aloud, the way you routinely announce procedure stimuli to patients or explain to patients what will happen to them during their procedure or office visit. Note if you use negative suggestions and compose alternative wording.

CHAPTER 9

Providing a Sense of Control

Case 9.1 The Handbag Holdup

A patient was brought from the ward into the procedure suite for placement of a large vein catheter. The patient was very apprehensive and agitated. She reiterated again and again that she was worried about her handbag. She conceded that she didn't need anything out of it at the moment, but was, nevertheless, very concerned about not having it. She had asked the personnel on her 5th floor ward to lock the handbag away safely for her before she left with the transporter for the procedure suite. Hoping to ease the patient's concern, a member of the procedure team called the attending ward nurse, who assured the team member that the handbag was still locked away safely in the ward. The procedure team member passed the word on to the patient, but the information and assurance did nothing to lessen the patient's distress; if anything, the fidgeting escalated. There was no objective reason—at least from the procedure team's perspective—why the patient should need her handbag at this time. The patient, however, continued to be very anxious. Out of consideration, a procedure nurses ran up to the ward, picked up the handbag, carried it into the procedure suite, and placed it under the patient's knees. The patient relaxed immediately—even without handling or looking into the handbag—she was content. Handbag and knees were covered under sterile drapes and the catheter placement proceeded uneventfully. ***Case Notes, E. Lang***

What This Case Illustrates Patients characteristically perceive that the usual control they have over themselves is abruptly and severely limited once they enter a medical environment. Patients may respond to this dread of loss of control by "testing" how much control they have left. A common test is to make requests or state needs to medical staff. When medical professionals make efforts to fulfill those needs—even when the request seems out of place—their supportive action validates the patient and provides him or her with a sense of control. Arguing or rationalizing about the legitimacy of patient's needs typically is counterproductive and makes things worse.

Control as a Moderator of Stress

Most of what has been published about the effect of control or lack thereof relates to chronic work-related challenges. Karasek[1] postulated a Job-Demand-Control Model in the 1970's, which was then expanded to a Job-Demand-Control-Support Model.[2; 3] Extensive studies on the topic suggest that high demand/low control situations adversely affect health and wellbeing and that providing a higher level of control to the situation can buffer some of these effects.[2; 3] Experiments in which people are intentionally placed under acute stress with controllable and uncontrollable stressors are harder to find. In a study in which volunteers were subjected to loud noise, volunteers who were given no control of the noise experienced higher elevations of stress hormones and greater activation of the sympathetic nervous system than did volunteers who were given some control of the noise.[4] In 1971, Ervin Staub and colleagues published a study in which volunteers received electric shocks of successively increasing intensity on their forearms.[5] Subjects who were given control over a switch that affected the intensity of the shocks experienced significantly higher thresholds for pain and were able to endure shocks for longer periods compared to subjects who received the exact same type of shocks but had no control over the switch. More modern experiments with animals produced similar results. Experiments where rats were able or unable to control shocks to their tail suggest that provision of control reduces stress-induced adverse effects through inhibition of neural activity in the brainstem.[6]

Requests as Means of Establishing a Sense of Control

In the modern medical setting, patients have some, albeit limited, control. They may choose a physician or facility, refuse treatment, or demand that a procedure or test be terminated; and the requests will be honored—within the limits of safety and bureaucratic confines. Once in a high tech medical or surgical suite, however, a sense of lack of control may become pervasive and may contribute to their anxiety.[7] It is important that patients' request are taken seriously in this situation because response to requests has a far reach. How successful the medical team is in meeting a patient's requests during a medical encounter turns out to be a major determinant of that patient's satisfaction with his or her overall medical experience.[8] Making requests may be the only avenue patients find open to them to prove—or to test—their control capacity. We often encounter requests from patients when they are brought into the procedure room which, on first hearing, may seem unreasonable or out of place—as in the case 9.1, "The Handbag Holdup." Nevertheless, we have come to take these requests very seriously; and have made the idea of providing the perception of control an integral component of our teaching of empathy and also a necessary part of implementing successful hypnotic intervention. We have identified the following key strategies for bringing about the perception of control in patients:

- Give a swift response to simple requests. Example: If the patient complains of chill, don't challenge the sensation; instead quickly provide a blanket just out of the warmer.
- Solicit the patient's wishes. Example: Use sentences such as, "Please let us know at any time what we can do to make you more comfortable."
- If fulfilling requests verbatim would jeopardize safety, come up with a substitute. The substitute should validate the patient's need and reflect your sincere efforts to provide the essence of the patient's request. You may need to be creative in finding an alternative to what the patient wants. Once a patient has tested your willingness to satisfy a request, he or she will likely be more cooperative.

Sometimes compromise is called for when responding to patients' requests. We frequently recall a case of a diabetic patient who had become enraged because of a pre-procedure exchange with one of the personnel. The repercussion of that exchange was that the patient insisted on having food "NOW!" or he was "Outta here!" Quickly weighing our options, we presented him with the only food available, which was an attractive box of candies we had been presented with the day before. Deliberately, the patient picked a small chocolate figure, placed it on his chest and held it there for the next hour during the procedure—without eating it.[9] Our thoughts at that time were as follows: First, we knew this patient from before and were well aware that his threat to leave was real, and that his leaving would place his ischemic leg at greater risk. Second, one piece of candy—even if he had kept it in his mouth or swallowed it—would not have affected his diabetes in a way that was beyond our ability to control. One must always use discretion in cases such as this where you see no easy solution at first. Offering a tradeoff is often successful. Usually, a mutually agreeable compromise can be suggested.

JOURNAL ENTRY 9.1

The Perfect Stitch

A patient was to undergo change of a bile tube. She had experienced several exchanges before and the tube was sutured to the skin to prevent its falling out. The suture consists of a nylon thread, which is affixed to the skin with a loop and then tightly wrapped around the tube a few times, closed with a knot, and finally cut to leave about 1-cm long ends sticking out. The patient agreed that the procedure was to be done under hypnosis; but no matter how hard Dr. Laser worked, the patient did not go into trance. Each time the induction failed, Dr. Laser asked, "What's stopping you?" The patient did not answer. Dr. Laser's question and the patient's silence went on for three passes—one after each induction attempt. Then the patient raised her head, and said, "I don't want to tell you what to do, but, Dr. Lang, the stitches scratched me last time. Can you turn them the other way?" Dr. Lang replied, "Of course, you are the expert." "Shall I turn them this way?" Dr. Lang asked, as she placed the loop on the top rather than the side of the tube. "Yes!" the woman replied, "that will be better." This was not just an idle hope. We had learned that the patient made patchwork quilts for a living, and she knows how to sew properly to get specific results.

Journal Notes, E. Laser

We have found that in cases such as "The Perfect Stitch," where induction attempts repeatedly fail, that the patient usually has an underlying issue that is bothering her or him. It is not always easy to fish out the reason. After she spoke and resolved her worry, the patient was compliant and went into trance easily. This case illustrates how doctor and patient sometimes need to sort things out between them, and when they do, the resistance usually disappears.

JOURNAL ENTRY 9.2

A Coffee and a Smoke

A patient was scheduled in the Radiology department for the removal of gallstones through the skin using instruments guided by X-Rays and an endoscope—a procedure that typically takes a few hours. It was in the afternoon, and the patient really, really wanted "a coffee and a smoke." Since patients are typically left without food after midnight for these procedures and also do not receive fluids by mouth for 6 hours before, one could easily sympathize with his cravings. Giving him a cup of coffee for which "he could have killed for" was not an option because drinking on the procedure table could have risked him regurgitating the fluid into his lungs. We couldn't fulfill his actual requests so we provided him with the essence of his desired experiences. We brewed a fresh pot of coffee in the lounge, and soaked a 4x4 gauze with enough of the coffee to wet his lips. Our efforts satisfied his yearning for coffee. He was very pleased and requested only one additional coffee swab "drink" later. The smoking request was even easier to fulfill. We promised to let him smoke in hypnosis, which he now happily accepted, and, indeed, he did smoke—in his imagination, for the whole 2 hours. ***Journal Notes, E. Lang***

JOURNAL ENTRY 9.3

Puppy Love—The Best Medicine

One day when my husband came to the hospital to meet me for lunch, he told me of an incredible sight he had just witnessed. A team of nurses had brought a patient in her bed to the side entrance of the hospital. The patient must have been quite sick judging by the number of IV poles and pumps that had been transported with her. On a signal, a car drove up to the entrance, parked, and out stepped a man holding a small dog. It was apparently the patient's dog. Someone held the little dog up to the patient and both patient and dog were exuberant with joy. I just couldn't imagine any medicine or therapy that might have lifted the patient's spirits more than this simple reunion. From the medical staff's perspective, it would have been so much easier to tell this patient that animals are not allowed into the hospital and that she can't see her puppy while she is here. I'm sure the patient loved seeing and touching her beloved pet and I am also convinced that the patient felt assured that she had not lost all control by entering the hospital. ***Journal Notes, E. Lang***

Some patient requests are simple; others take a bit of creativity and actual effort to satisfy. The effort is well worth the reward—aiding the patient's comfort and wellbeing by providing the perception of control for the patient.

Key Points to Remember

- Lack of control has undesirable effects on health and wellbeing and enhances the adverse effects of stress.
- Once patients enter the medical high tech environment or any procedure area, the sense of lack of control can be pervasive and contribute to their anxiety.
- Making requests may be the only avenue patients find open to them to prove—or to test—their control capacity.
- Although some requests can't be met verbatim for safety reasons, all efforts should be made to either comply with a request or come up with a substitute that will validate the patient's need and provide the essence of the patient's request.

- You must always use discretion in cases where you see no easy solution at first. Offering a tradeoff is often successful.
- In cases where suggestions for relaxation or induction of hypnosis induction fail, the patient usually has an underlying issue that is bothering her or him.

Opportunities to Practice

- Notice what patients ask for in stressful situations and observe what happens when you fulfill their requests.
- Think of what requests patients in your area often express, but don‘t receive, and come up with creative alternatives that provide the essence of the experience without risks.

CHAPTER 10

Encouraging Actions, Not Praising Actors

Case 10.1 Chain of Encouragement

The Patient Sedation Without Medication workshop that Drs. Lang and Laser were providing for a group of technologists, nurses, and physicians was presented in modules. During the Rapport Module, Drs. Lang and Laser introduced an exercise to workshop participants by telling them that they were going to give one another a statement of encouragement to inspire continuation of specific behavior. Immediately there was loud resistance. A number of participants voiced the belief that having to quickly think up and confer a compliment on colleagues out of the blue would be insincere and counter productive. The protestors insisted that they would perceive such a compliment directed to them as either "brown-nosing" or "leg-pulling." Dr. Laser calmed their fears somewhat by explaining that the goal of the exercise was not to make a global quality assessment to label the person, such as "you are a great nurse." Dr. Laser went on to tell them that in contrast, this statement of encouragement was to take the form of an expression of acknowledgement and appreciation for specific behavior that the person was doing or had done and which the bestower of the encouragement personally admired, and/or for which he or she was sincerely grateful.

Although still fairly reluctant, the group agreed to proceed. Dr. Laser asked participants to note the person on their right and to begin to identify specific positive behaviors of that person to encourage. Dr. Lang identified one person to start a "chain of encouragement." Dr. Lang asked that person to turn to the colleague sitting to his right and give encouragement in the form of a few words of appreciation for something specific the colleague was generally doing or had done. Next, Dr. Lang asked the just-encouraged-person to turn to the person to her right and say a few words of appreciation to encourage that person. Thus, Dr. Laser pointed out the encouragement chain would progress around the circle with each encouraged person, in turn, looking to the person to his or her right and saying a few words of specific appreciation to encourage the mentioned behavior. The process would continue, she explained, until the circle was complete and everyone had the opportunity to give and to receive an encouraging statement of appreciation for specific actions.

Although many of the participants had worked years together on the same procedure team—some for more than 10 years—and had spent innumerable days and nights on cases together, rarely had any of them encouraged specific behavior of a teammate by expressing appreciation of that behavior and sharing what that teammate's contribution meant to them personally. One technologist noted how much help and comfort it was to him, being a new team member, to have a more senior technologist mentor him. A nurse expressed how the calm demeanor of one of her colleagues when they were both under stress had helped the nurse understand that the patient's anger was fear based and was not a personal affront to her. Another team member expressed appreciation for a colleague who had taken over some administrative billing work, which indirectly helped several people to keep their jobs. A technologist thanked another for having taken, despite personal inconvenience, a holiday night call, and how doing that had given the encouraging technologist an opportunity to visit an ailing relative and how much that had meant to her. Someone expressed appreciation for a person who had stood up for colleagues in a time of crisis, which had helped to keep the team together. As the circle progressed, people became more and more moved and deeply touched by what was said. It seemed that years of mutual respect and gratitude surfaced that, in general, had not been clearly expressed before. The exercise was a success. All of the participants expressed how motivating it felt to receive this specific encouragement. ***Case Notes, E. Lang***

What This Case Illustrates Many people are uncomfortable with and even suspect statements bestowed under the guise of praise that slap a label on them as a whole e.g. "great doctor," "smart woman," "good patient." In contrast, having their specific behavior acknowledged in the form of statements of appreciation for that behavior makes most people feel valued and encourages them to continue their efforts with confidence. Acknowledging and expressing appreciation for efforts made are two of the mainstays of giving encouragement that will motivate further positive actions.

Encouragement Versus Praise

Medical procedures go smoother and quicker when patients cooperate. Demanding that people behave in a certain way rarely works, but encouraging them to do so usually does.[1] Encouragement is most effective in an environment of mutual respect. Respect cannot be demanded. It must be earned. It can emanate from a relationship when rapport is established and the patient's problems as well as their efforts are acknowledged, honored, and validated. In our work, we use encouraging statements to establish an atmosphere of mutual respect and to promote specific patient behaviors that will help us help the patient.

Temporary stress or unfortunate habit leads some practitioners to resort to warnings and threats to get the behavior they want. They might say, "If you keep breathing like this, we will have to do the films all over again." Or, " Please listen to me! I've told you several times not to move at the critical moment, you won't be able to complete the test if you continue moving like this." This approach seldom works and often makes matters worse. Even when the patient complies, the relationship is damaged and the patient's willingness to consent to subsequent medical encounters may suffer.

When intending to encourage the patient toward certain behaviors, it's important not to confuse encouragement with praise that assesses and labels the person as a whole. Unlike such praise, encouragement emphasizes the deed, not the doer; the action, not the actor. When you encourage, you inspire and motivate the person to certain behaviors. You cheer on his or her efforts. For example, because having the patient hold still is crucial for the success of many procedures or parts of procedures, we acknowledge and encourage the effort to hold still when we see it—or even when we see the hint of an attempt at it. We might say, "Your holding this position so still is helping the procedure go very well."

In contrast, the emphasis of whole person praise is to judge and to label the person as a whole. Typical statements of such praise include: "You're such a good patient." "You're an awesome technician." "You're wonderful." In praise interactions, the person giving praise is often perceived as the authority, the person who must be pleased. Psychologists Jennifer Henderlong of Reed College and Mark Lepper of Stanford University performed an extensive review and found that praise that focuses on the person can undermine motivation in children if the children believe that their recognition had mainly resulted from their success in pleasing the authority.[(2)]

Most of the current literature addressing encouragement and praise, such as Henderlong and Lepper's review, as well as Don Dinkmeyer and Rudolf Dreikurs' much revered book, *Encouraging Children to Learn*[1] has been established with children and adolescents in an educational setting. Dr. Laser, who is well versed in these concepts from her work in the education field, perceived that the teacher/student relationship was, in important ways, comparable to that of practitioner/patient. As a result, we were very successful in transferring the principles behind promoting encouragement in lieu of judgmental, labeling praise into the clinical arena.

The literature, as well as our experience, reveals that one of the major downsides of praise is that it discourages self-evaluation. If the patient sets high personal standards for himself or herself, and the practitioner praises behavior that does not yet reach these standards, the patient might feel insulted. On the other hand, once the practitioner has introduced the element of praise, the patient may start to rely solely on praise for validation. The result is that even when the patient is feeling proud of his or her own performance, but praise is not given, the patient may loose confidence and self-esteem. In general, praising—judging and labeling—a person may make him or her feel demeaned and could give rise to overt or covert anger, which can destroy rapport, discourage desired patient behaviors, and, ultimately, sabotage the practitioner's goals.

Offering praise risks being perceived as phony, particularly when it is highly effusive or overly general.[3] When a person does not believe such praise he or she may even behave oppositely just to show that he or she is not correctly labeled.[4] People will discount and may even be angered by praise that they feel is insincere or is offered by an evaluator whom they feel lacks the appropriate knowledge necessary to judge them.[2] Such was Dr. Laser's experience when a sincere, casual compliment she gave was misconstrued.

JOURNAL ENTRY 10.1

The Good Teacher

I remember a time I was asked to observe a teacher and her class in her classroom. I sat quietly, and as I left the room, I said, "You are a good teacher." To my utter surprise, the teacher reported me and my compliment to the supervisor, who called me in for a chat. Upon careful review of the incident, I realized that the teacher resented my pronouncement that she was a "good" teacher. The explanation of her rancor—which she relayed to the supervisor—was summed up in one sentence, "How would she (Me) know what was or was not 'good' teaching." Because the teacher knew I was not a classroom teacher at her level, she, apparently, did not value my assessment of the quality of her teaching. I tried to learn from this; it has remained in my memory as a teaching aid for illustrating the pitfalls of praise, even when sincerely given. ***Journal Notes, E. Laser***

As Dr. Laser's experience illustrates, even a simple compliment can backfire when the person has a standard for him- or herself that is higher than what impressed the person giving the complement or when the complemented person does not value the label given in the compliment. In one of her "Rhymes with Orange" comic strips, Hilary Price brings this point home by showing a dog on the psychotherapist's couch complaining "Sure it's always "good dog," but is it ever "great dog?"

Articulating Encouragement

It is so easy to forget to express appreciation for the contribution that friends, colleagues, and patients make that improve our lives. We tend to take these for granted or may just assume the others know how we feel about their efforts. Opportunities for making encouraging statements to patients abound in medical settings. One might just think of what it takes for patients to be at the hospital at 7 AM in the morning without eating; perhaps having had to travel long distances, which required getting up in the middle of the night; or lying on a procedure table for hours. Just acknowledging this effort and accomplishment can go far in eliciting further collaboration from the patient. Encouragement validates the patient's efforts and establishes a partnership necessary for the desirable outcome of a medical encounter. Encouraging statements should contain three elements:

- A description of specific behavior
- An expression of your appreciation of the behavior
- An explanation of how the behavior contributes to a beneficial outcome

Note that expressions of appreciation basically involve some mix of approval, admiration, and gratitude. Following are some encouragement examples: "Thank you for holding your breath so long; your not moving made it possible to get a really good picture." "How wonderful that you brought all the charts with you. They will help us coordinate your care and help all of us shape a more effective care plan for you." "I noticed how hard you worked at this and I admire your persistence. Your not giving up makes it possible for us to complete the procedure much faster."

There has to be something your patient is doing right. Think about what it is and make at least one encouraging statement during the encounter.

Just as important as learning to give encouragement appropriately, is learning to accept encouragement. It is okay to give and it is okay to receive encouragement. When you receive encouragement, don't nix it. Don't say "oh that was nothing" or worse, "no problem," since doing so will invalidate the valiant effort of the person offering encouragement. A simple "thank you." will do just fine if you can't find other words.

Key Points to Remember

- Many people are uncomfortable with and even suspect of statements bestowed under the guise of praise that slaps a label on them as a whole.
- Having their specific behavior acknowledged in the form of statements of appreciation for that behavior makes most people feel validated and encourages them to continue their efforts with confidence.
- Demanding that patients behave in a certain way rarely works, but encouraging them to do so usually does.
- Unlike judgmental, labeling praise, encouragement emphasizes the deed, not the doer; the action, not the actor.
- One of the major downsides of praise is that it discourages self-evaluation.
- Encouraging statements should contain three elements: A description of specific behavior, an expression of your appreciation of the behavior, and an explanation of how the behavior contributes to a beneficial outcome.
- Expressions of appreciation basically involve some mix of approval, admiration, and gratitude.

Opportunities to Practice

- Give each of your next 10 patient a few words of encouragement (not praise) and notice the reaction and how the subsequent encounter evolves.
- Think of a contribution that your colleagues or friends have made to your life and that you want to acknowledge. Think of what you are going to say. Remember, the deed, not the doer; the action, not the actor. Be sure to include what their behavior accomplished. Write it out if it will help. Then just say it.

PART III

CHAPTER 11

Overview and Elements of Hypnosis

Case 11.1 The H-Word

When offering sedation without medication in the early 1990's, many of our trainees were not yet ready to use the word *hypnosis* to describe the process. One day, one of the nurses was leading a patient down the long hallway towards the MRI scanner and talking about the upcoming examination. The patient was anxious and uncertain of what to expect. When offered a relaxation exercise, he countered that when he tries to relax he just tenses up. The nurse offered him alternative explanations of how she might help him. She said she "could guide him in imagery," he didn't want any part of that. She suggested that he could, "go on a magic journey in his mind," he said he had a poor imagination. The nurse offered, "visualization," he said no, it won't work. She explained, "It would be like day dreaming," he didn't do that either. Somewhat exasperated she then asked him, "Don't you ever have a fantasy?" His eyes lighted up, "Oh sure, a fantasy, yes, I do." By that time they had arrived at the scanner and she told him firmly, "Okay, you go in there now and have a fantasy, and have it in color!" He confidently walked into the scanner room. An invitation to have a fantasy on his own—in color yet—was all he needed to focus his mind and take his attention away from the noise and workings of the MRI machine. He completed the whole scan sequence without incident and apparently without discomfort. ***Case Notes, E. Lang***

What This Case Illustrates The self-hypnotic state is a natural phenomenon that everyone is familiar with but may call by a different name. It is the process that's important, not the label term.

Goals of the Use of Hypnosis for Patient Sedation

As you begin Part III of *Patient Sedation Without Medication,* it's important to zero in on the scope and purpose of the presentation of hypnotic techniques you are about to encounter. These chapters will not teach you how to exert mind control—as depicted in scary/funny movies where the villain stares a maiden into his spell. You will find no lessons here in how to make patients or colleagues cluck like chickens, nor guidelines for how to amuse yourself and others by performing a stage show. What this part of *Patient Sedation Without Medication* will offer you are adjuncts that you can incorporate into your daily professional tasks to help you help your patients through a stressful situation. The extra benefit to you is that the act of your carrying out these techniques with patients will also reduce your own stress.

You probably are already using techniques that you think may help your patients. The information presented here can help you clarify and evaluate those techniques; and help you decide which you can build upon, which may not be what they seem, and which you may want to reshape or no longer use. Also, you will learn new approaches that can bring a positive outcome.

Completing the lessons in *Patient Sedation Without Medication* will not make you a hypnotherapeutic psycholoanalyst, and your role and purpose as proposed by this book is not to provide family therapy or attempt to fix patients' underlying problems with life, relationships, or psychopathology. The goal that this book is designed to meet is that of helping you be able to help your patients complete a medical test or procedure safely and without unnecessary medication, which too often carry risks for patients. Another benefit of procedure hypnosis is that it makes patients hemodynamically more stable and thus, reduces complication rates.[1; 2]

Furthermore, *Patient Sedation Without Medication* is designed to increase your comfort and efficacy in your work with patients by guiding you to channel your empathy in ways that do not hurt and only help the patient, which will enhance your enjoyment of work.[2] You will also receive more positive feedback from your patients.

Overview of Hypnosis

Hypnosis is a state of attentive receptive concentration that helps patients to explore their own capacity to interact with a painful or uncomfortable situation.[3] If you have ever become so absorbed in a movie, book, or computer game that you forgot about a painful body part, you have experienced such a state. Hypnosis is not something done to a person, rather all hypnosis is essentially self-hypnosis.[4] In the same way you would not become fully absorbed in a book or movie you don't like, another person cannot hypnotize you against your will. The subject of hypnosis is always in control and free to accept and use the suggestions offered or to ignore or reject them outright. So we must disappoint anyone who may have thought to acquire Svengali-like mind controlling powers by reading this book.

The hypnotic process includes *trance*. In trance, the mind no longer keeps in awareness what is happening around in the periphery.[4] It is easy to go into trance, and you've no doubt done it: you may look out of the kitchen window and get lost in thought forgetting the pot on the stove until it boils over; you may start to think of something while in a class or conversation, and when you are suddenly expected to give an answer, you have no clue of what the topic is, much less what the other person just asked you. These are examples of trance, but are not hypnosis. *Hypnosis* is trance with content and purpose. Therefore, all hypnosis includes trance, but not all trance is hypnosis.

There are essentially two paths to hypnosis. In formal hypnosis, a practitioner guides (induces) the patient to enter trance and then makes suggestions for a scenario (imagery), in which the patient might imagine him- or herself, in order to overcome challenges such as pain, anxiety, or worries. Once a patient has been guided in formal hypnosis, he or she can then use the ritualized suggestions of trance induction to enter self-hypnosis without the practitioner even being there. The other path to hypnosis is specifically referred to as self-hypnosis; through it one can enter hypnosis just on one's own without formal training or anybody else's input.

JOURNAL ENTRY 11.1

Escape in the Trickling Stream

In talking with an associate about the instinctive quality of hypnosis, I recalled how—without knowing what it was—I used it when I was a child and had to go to the dentist. Dentists at the time didn't use Novocain unless perhaps for a root canal. I found out quickly that doing complex multiplications—say 17 x 59—in my head did help divert my attention from the sound and the smell and the pain of the drilling. If the dental appointment fell in springtime, I would let my mind wander along the flowers in a huge blooming magnolia tree right outside the dental office window. My associate said that thinking about it, she, too, remembers having instinctively used self-hypnosis—without any knowledge of the term or the process—to deal with dental appointments as a child. We remembered that both our dentists had a *spit sink*—a small round white porcelain basin next to the treatment chair. A thin stream of blue liquid poured from a tiny spigot along one side and swirled around and around in a diminishing spiral towards the center drain. She welcomed those moments of respite from the drilling when she was allowed to bend over the sink to spit. Seeing the tiny stream triggered memories of being at a small, barely trickling brook that emptied into a small pool with shade trees, moss, and watercress—an inviting and safe place she liked to visit. Back upright, as the drill whirred, she would picture being by the brook. The soft gurgle of the tiny spit-sink stream on its path from spigot to drain helped with the imagery. Her teeth needed to be worked on, but she could play by the brook. Spit sinks being long gone, and dental appoints still happening, my associate says she now finds imagery inspiration in the artificial banana tree and picture of a stylized parrot on the back wall of her current dentist's treatment room. Imagined jungle scenes and sounds now, quite naturally, push the dental work out of mind. ***Journal Notes, E. Lang***

The Process of Procedure Hypnosis

Hypnosis is a process. In the following chapters, you will be guided through that process. The first process element to consider is induction. *Induction* is the term used to describe the process of leading a patient into hypnosis or into a hypnotic trance. Hypnotic inductions often include suggestions for relaxation. While relaxation helps to experience hypnosis, relaxation or meditation exercises alone do not constitute hypnosis[(5)] In contradistinction to other forms of trance, there has to be a goal associated with the exercise to be hypnosis.[(6)] A goal might be a change in behavior, such as being less anxious; being able to complete a procedure; or being able to heal faster. Chapters 12, "Hypnosis by Script," and 13,

"Inductions Using Eye Fixation and Movements," offer specific techniques for induction. Some patients want to experience hypnosis, but try as they might, are unable to enter trance. Chapter 14, "Confusional Inductions," provides strategies for these patients for whom more traditional induction approaches are not successful in helping them into trance.

In addition to making their subconscious mind more open to suggestions, patients in hypnosis can communicate what their subconscious mind is revealing. They can do this without speaking by using the process element of ideomotor signals. *Ideomotor* refers to a subconscious idea being expressed as an involuntary or automatic motor signal. The automatic nodding of the head when hearing something one agrees with is a common example of ideomotor signals. Chapter 15, "Ideomotor Signals," explains how to set up and use the patient's ideomotor signals to communicate during the procedure.

Although patients can communicate without speaking, practitioners typically do speak, and what they say has power. A very important factor to consider in the process of hypnosis—or in being around patients in general—is language use. Patients in a medical setting often—just on their own—enter a state of hypnosis, and in so doing, become highly suggestive and receptive to what is said around them.[(7)] The language patients hear—the language you and others around the patient use—thus greatly affects the patient's experience. This is true whether you formally induce hypnosis or the patient has entered a state of self-hypnosis by him- or herself. Whatever you tell a patient in this state is called a *suggestion* and is an invitation for the subconscious mind to consider. You have already learned in chapter 8, "Avoiding Negative Suggestions," of the importance of keeping your words positive. In chapters 16, "Uses and Misuses of *Trying*," and 17, "Direct and Indirect Language," we provide more specifics of how to use language effectively during hypnosis.

The use of imagery is a mainstay element of procedure hypnosis. Imagery replaces a person's attention on the peripheral surroundings and concurrent reality with focus on past, future, or imagined content. Imagery can be experienced as being within one's body and being absorbed in the situation with all one's senses or from the viewpoint of an observer from a distant perspective. Techniques for assisting patients in use of imagery—including how to counter distressing imagery are detailed in Chapter 18, "Imagery."

Difficulties—often due to the ramifications of the medical procedure—can arise with the patient before and during procedure hypnosis. Anxiety is a common difficulty for patients who come for medical procedures. Chapter 19, "Managing Anxiety and Distress," explains ways to ease patient distress and anxiety both before and during the medical procedure, and offers strategies for dealing with anxiety that has assumed imagery in the patient's mind. Optimizing patients' pain relief is an everyday goal in any invasive medical procedure suite. The experience of pain is subjective. Chapter 20, "Managing Pain," explains that hypnosis helps with pain management in two ways: by taking the mind off what is hurting and by changing how the stimulus is processed in the brain. The chapter offers several approaches to pain management. Adverse physiological events are also common during medical procedures. Chapter 21, " Stabilizing Physiology," explains how to use the patient's subconscious mind to adjust blood pressure or other physiological factors that become an issue.

The final hypnosis process element is reorientation—the process at the end of patients' test or procedure of reorienting patients in hypnosis to their natural state of awareness. Chapter 22, "Reorientation," provides various methods of reorientation, discusses the phenomena of time distortion and posthypnotic amnesia, and offers strategies for making use of posthypnotic suggestions to help patients recover.

Offering Hypnosis to the Patient

Displaying rapid rapport skills does not require permission or explanation; hypnosis does. Although eventually the word may get around (and it happens quickly) that you offer procedure hypnosis and, therefore, some patients will soon specifically select your practice for that option; in the beginning, many, if not most, likely will not anticipate that you have hypnosis to offer. Although patients are much more open to mind-body techniques and holistic approaches than just 10 or 15 years ago, chances are still good that hypnosis may be a new concept or patients might have misconceptions about it that lean heavily toward the context of stage hypnosis and scary movies of mind-controlling monsters. Patients come to their medical appointments for a doctor visit or procedure, not a psychology session. They are typically somewhat frightened. Confronted with a frightened patient unaware and/or ill-informed about hypnosis along with your own reservations about a difficult procedure, you need to have considered beforehand how you will offer patient sedation without medication.

To make the proposition of applying what you have learned and giving the patients the choice to help themselves, you need to include the following basic pieces of information.

- Introduce the offer. Let the patient know, in terms he or she will easily understand that hypnosis is available. You might say, "One of the options we can offer you today to keep you comfortable during your procedure is _____ (hypnosis) (self-hypnosis) (relaxing techniques) (visualizing techniques) (taking an imaginary journey during the procedure)."
- Explain what the patient can expect from the experience. You might say, "It is just a form of

concentration, like reading a book or watching a movie, where one forgets one is reading a book or watching a movie and the world around you becomes less important. Have you had such an experience?" Most people will affirm that they have.

- Assure the patient that he or she will always be in control of the process. You might say, "I've explained that it's like getting lost in a book or a movie and you know that this only happens with a book or movie you like. So you remain fully in control. No one can be hypnotized against his or her will."
- Explain that extensive research has been done about procedure hypnosis and provide the evidence that what you have to offer is clinically tested. You might say, "We have used this successfully, and large clinical studies have shown that patients are more relaxed and have better outcomes with this process." Also add (if it is true), "I am experienced in guiding patients during their examination."
- After obtaining permission, you can ask the patient if he or she would like to use the technique you described. You might say, "Would you like to go on a journey? You know, your body has to be here, but you don't. Is there a place you always wanted to go? You even don't need to pack. If you want, we can go there right now."

Caution: There are specific circumstances when you should not use hypnosis. Specifically when working with a patient to relive abuse, rape, or any criminal event. Hypnosis in this setting may make the testimony of the person against the perpetrator in court inadmissible.[(8)] You should steer clear of offering hypnosis to patients with psychoses, in particular multiple personality disorder. For most patients, however, procedure hypnosis is a good choice. Although in a hypnotic trance, patients are able to communicate verbally, follow instructions, maintain their airway, control their breathing, and move into desired positioning during procedures. This is of great advantage as compared to subjecting patients to anesthesia or heavy medical sedation where cooperation in breath holding or adjustment of body position becomes difficult or impossible.

Key Points to Remember

- Trance is a natural phenomenon and common experience for which people use different words such as daydreaming, spacing out, being completely absorbed in a task, concentrating fully, being mesmerized, having a fantasy. It is the process that's important not the label term.
- Hypnosis is a state of attentive receptive concentration that helps patients to explore their own capacity to interact with a painful or uncomfortable situation.
- All hypnosis is essentially self-hypnosis, not something that is done to the patient, and the operator is only a guide helping patients help themselves.
- The subject of hypnosis is always in control of the process.
- Hypnosis is trance with content and purpose. Therefore, all hypnosis includes trance, but not all trance is hypnosis.
- While relaxation helps to experience hypnosis, relaxation or meditation exercises alone do not constitute hypnosis.
- Displaying rapid rapport skills does not require permission or explanation; hypnosis does.
- To make the proposition of applying what you have learned and giving the patients the choice to help themselves, you may want to include the following basic pieces

of information: introduce the offer, explain what to expect, assure the patient that he or she will be in control of the process, and explain that there is evidence for the effectiveness and safety of the process in this setting.

- Patients are able to communicate and follow instruction in hypnosis, which helps them cooperate during procedures.

Opportunities to Practice

- Read again script 1.1, "Experiencing Confidence," to experience hypnosis yourself and prepare yourself for learning the hypnotic techniques in the subsequent chapters.
- For now, hold off from using hypnotic techniques with your patients until you have read all of Part III.

CHAPTER 12
Hypnosis by Script

Case 12.1 In Search of a Script

In the early 1990s, Dr. Lang's research and clinical group was getting ready to start its first large scale prospective randomized controlled hypnosis trial, which targeted patients having interventional radiological procedures. The study was funded by the National Institutes of Health (NIH), and the reviewers required that the trial use methods that any compassionate healthcare provider could master. Lang's group was cautioned to not include complicated methods that only a virtuoso in hypnotic technique could apply. What's more, the methods had to be clearly defined and identifiable if one were to watch a video of the case.

Dr. Lang's group prepared a manual that defined all the elements of hypnosis and all the rapid rapport components to be tested in the trial. To further ensure standardization, the group agreed that a script would be used to guide patients into hypnosis and through their procedures, which included catheter manipulations either in their blood vessels or kidneys and ureters.

Induction is the term used to describe the process of leading a patient into hypnosis or into a hypnotic trance. Inductions involve the practitioner making ritualized suggestions to the patient. These ritualized suggestions had to be spelled out in a script that all investigators would use. Dr. Lang's group had tried out several scripts and inductions and found them unsatisfactory. The available short induction, "Your eyes won't close until your inner mind gives you permission," required advanced skills and came across as "weird" to some of the research assistants. There were classic hypnotic inductions available that didn't have those shortcomings, but they had an inherent problem of their own—length. Classic hypnotic inductions were quite long and in the hectic medical environment, very likely to be interrupted before they could be concluded. The classic inductions varied in content. Some inductions included relaxation sequences; others counting numbers backward, and still others had patients stepping down a set of stairs. Dr. Lang recalls the last case in which she used the descent from stair 10 downward. She guided the patient down from step 10 to step 9, and was at step 8 when a relief nurse walked into the room, went straight to the patient and introduced herself loudly breaking the incipient trance. Dr. Lang began down again from step 10. This time she got to step five when the physician performing the medical procedure yelled a command. The induction sequence was broken again. Dr. Lang wondered whether to keep walking the patient down from step 5 or starting again at step 10. Disenchanted with the process, Dr. Lang decided that this was the last time she would use an induction that employed walking stairs, or counting numbers backward, or anything else that required a lengthy sequence so susceptible to interruption.

Dr. Lang listed the features that she required in a script: The script must be relatively immune to interruptions; the induction should be quick to apply; and, if needed, easily repeatable. It must address fears early on and in a straightforward way, release the patient's imagery without resistance, have provisions for management of pain and anxiety, and conclude with a simple reorientation. Dr. Lang brought her concerns about available induction scripts along with a list of the script characteristics that her research required to Dr. David Spiegel, Professor of Psychiatry and Behavioral Sciences at Stanford University, who was a consultant on the study. At the conclusion of their discussion, Dr. Spiegel picked up his Dictaphone and out came the script that was used from then on in the study. With some minor modification and additions, this script, referred to as the *Study Script,* (Script 12.1 printed below) has stood the test of time. It has been used with hundreds of patients in the trials and clinical practice with great success. ***Case Notes, E. Lang***

What This Case Illustrates The use of scripts for induction and guidance through hypnosis can be efficient and ensure consistency. Care must be taken to compose suitable scripts from the wide array of available script elements. Making a list of the script characteristics that your situation requires will help you select or create an efficacious script for your purpose.

Use of Scripts

As you begin applying rapid hypnotic techniques, you may find it is easiest to use a script. Scripts can allay both the patient's misconceptions about hypnosis, that is, putting them under the control of an individual's momentary whim, and the practitioner's concerns about finding the right words and affecting a smooth presentation. The sight of the practitioner sitting down with a script tends to comfort the patient, taking away notions of capricious power and hocus-pocus.

You should never forgo using a script because you think it lessens your professionalism. There is no shame in reading from a script. Dr. Lang—even after many years of clinical practice—still often reads from the script described in case 12.1, "In Search of a Script," or from other scripts when working with patients. Over time, reading from scripts helps you become fluent in the language of hypnosis and more at ease in guiding patients—with or without a script. For professionals working in teams, scripts have another advantage; scripts help establish a common language and facilitate the handing off of the patient—along with the script—among team members if the practitioner needs to leave the procedures room while the hypnosis is in progress.

The remaining chapters in Part III of this book contain more scripts and script segments. The Script Appendix at the end of the book lists all of the scripts and script segments contained in *Patient Sedation Without Medication*. You can adapt the sample scripts and mix and match segments to craft your own scripts to meet the particular needs of your practice, style, and situation at hand. Scripts at a minimum should include the following components: induction, immunization against noise and unhelpful suggestions, pertinent suggestions, anchoring in a safe place, and a reorientation to the waking state. Each of these points will be illustrated and explained in this chapter. We begin with the modified Study Script Dr. David Spiegel developed for Dr. Lang's group. The script is presented first in its entirety and, in the following section titled Commentary on the Study Script, we analyze and comment on the script's specific components.

Script 12.1 The Study Script

We want you to help us to help you to learn a concentration exercise to help you get through the procedure more comfortably. It can be a way to help your body be more comfortable through the procedure and also deal with any discomfort that may come up during the procedure. It is just a form of concentration, like getting so caught up in a movie or a good book that you forget you are watching a movie or reading a book.

Now you may be interested to learn how you can use your imagination to enter a state of focused attention and physical relaxation. If you hear sounds or noises in the room, just use these to deepen your experience. And use only the suggestions that are helpful for you. There are a lot of ways to relax, but here is one simple way:

On *one,* you can do one thing—look up.

On *two,* two things, slowly close your eyes and take a deep breath.

On *three,* three things, breathe out, relax your eyes, and let your body float.

Good. Just imagine your whole body floating, floating right through the table, with each breath deeper and easier. Right now imagine that you are floating somewhere safe and comfortable, in a bath, a lake, a hot tub, or just floating in space, with each breath deeper and easier. Just notice how with each breath you let a little more tension out of your body as you let your whole body float, safe and comfortable; each breath deeper and easier. Good, now with your eyes closed and remaining in this state of concentration, please describe for me how your body is feeling right now. Where do you imagine yourself being? What is it like? Can you smell the air? Can you see what is around you? Good. Now this is your safe and pleasant place to be and you can use it in a sense to play a trick on the doctors *(or this whole procedure).* Your body has to be here, but you don't. So just spend your time being somewhere you would rather be.

Now, if there is some discomfort, and there may be some with the procedure as they prepare you and insert the line, or as you feel the dye entering your body, there is no point in fighting it. You can admit it, but then transform that sensation. If you feel some discomfort, you might find it helpful to make that part of your body to feel warmer, as if you were in a bath. Or cooler—if that is more comfortable—as if you had ice or snow on that part of your body. This warmth and coolness becomes a protective filter between you and the pain.

If you have any discomfort right now, imagine that you are applying a hot pack or that you are putting snow or ice on it and see what it feels like. Develop the sense of warm or cool or delicious tingling numbness to filter the hurt out of the pain.

With each breath, breathe deeper and easier, your body is floating, filter the hurt out of the pain.

Now, again with your eyes closed and remaining in the state of concentration, describe what you are feeling right now.

(Option 1) ***If patient is at his or her safe and comfortable place—reinforce it. Say:***

What is it like now? What do you see around you? What are you doing?

(Option 2) ***If patient is in pain—address it. Say:***

The pain is there but see if you can add coolness or more warmth or make it lighter or make it heavier.

(Option 1) ***If patient is no longer in pain, say:***

Good. Continue to focus on those sensations.

(Option 2) ***If patient is still in pain, say:***

Focus on sensations in another part of your body. Now rub your fingertips together and notice all of the delicate sensations in your fingertips and see how much you can observe about what it feels like to rub your thumb and forefingers together. How do you feel now?

(Option 1) ***If patient is not in pain, say:***

Good. Continue to focus on these sensations.

(Option 2) ***If patient is still in pain, say:***

Now imagine yourself being at ______ (patient's safe place) where you said you felt relaxed and comfortable. What is it like now? What is the temperature? What do you see around you?

(Option 3) ***If patient states that he or she is worried—address it. Say:***

Okay, your main job right now is to help your body feel comfortable so we will talk about what is worrying you. But first, no matter what we discuss, concentrate on your body floating. So let's get the floating back into your body. Imagine that you are in this favorite spot and when you are ready let me know by nodding your head; and then we will talk about what is worrying you. But remember no matter what we discuss, concentrate on your body floating and feel safe and comfortable.

So what is worrying you? *(Discuss)*

How do you feel now?

(Option 1) ***If patient is no longer worried, say:***

Good. Now continue to concentrate on your body floating, and feel safe and comfortable in your favorite place.

(Option 2) ***If patient is still worried, say:***

Okay, picture in your mind a screen like a movie screen, TV screen or a piece of clear blue sky. First you might see a pleasant scene on it. Now picture a large piece of blue screen divided in half. All right. Now on the left half, picture what you are worrying about on the screen. Now on the right half of the screen, picture what you will do about it, or what you would recommend someone else do about it. Keep your body floating. And if you are worrying about the outcome, okay admit it to yourself, but your body does not have to get uptight about it. You may, but your body does not have to.

Good. You know that whatever happens there is always something you can do. But for now just concentrate on keeping your body floating and feeling safe and comfortable.

From time to time throughout the procedure, say:

If you feel any sense of discomfort, you are welcome to let me know about it. You may use the filter to filter the hurt out of the pain, but by all means let me know and I will do what I can to help you with it as well. Whatever you do, just keep your body floating and concentrate on being in the place where you feel safe and comfortable.

When the procedure is finished, say:

Okay, the procedure is completed now. We are going to formally leave this state of concentration by counting backwards from three to one. On *three* get ready, on *two* with your eyes closed roll up your eyes, and on *one* let your eyes open and take a deep breath and let it out. That will be the end of the formal exercise, but when you come out of it, you will still have the feeling of comfort that you felt during it. Ready, three, two, one.

If the patient opens the eyes, say:

Take a deep breath, and feel refreshed and proud about having helped yourself through this procedure.

If the patient hasn't followed, say:

Three—get ready. *Two*—with your eyes closed, roll up your eyes. *One*—let your eyes open and take a deep breath, and feel refreshed and proud about having helped yourself through this procedure. ***End of Script 12.1***

Commentary on the Study Script

Specific parts of the Study Script are analyzed below. Extracts from the Study Script text appear in italic type. Discussion and relevant commentary of each extraction follow in roman type.

> *We want you to help us to help you to learn a concentration exercise to help you to get through the procedure more comfortably. You could even say, We want to help you so that you can help us to help you to learn a concentration exercise to help you to get through the procedure more comfortably.*

A little confusing, isn't it? This sentence is an example of the confusional induction technique, which is discussed in chapter 14, "Confusional Inductions." When the conscious mind becomes confused, it becomes less able to control the subconscious mind, which then has a better opportunity to open itself to upcoming suggestions. The introductory sentence above may also illustrate why it might be easier to read from a script rather than attempting this sentence from memory.

> *It is just a form of concentration, like getting so caught up in a movie or a good book that you forget you are watching a movie or reading a book.*

At this point you may even ask the patient, "Can you recall such an experience?" Most people will affirm that they have.

For patients who appear uneasy and concerned about mind control, you can help ally their fears by expanding the "good book or movie" analogy through statements similar to the one described in chapter 11, "Introduction to Hypnosis": "And as you know this only happens with a book or movie you like. Otherwise you would close the book or change the channel on TV or turn it off all together. You are always fully in control."

If you hear sounds or noises in the room, just use these to deepen your experience.

The medical procedure environment will have noises. People talk, the phone may ring, pagers may go off, perhaps a helicopter lands on the building, or a truck drives by. You want to reduce the risk of those noises startling or distracting the patient. Immunization against noise is critical. Dr. Lang, for example, helps make patients immune to the loud snap of the biopsy gun by demonstrating the sound (while holding the device out of sight from the patient). At the sound, Dr. Lang tells the patient, "Every time you hear this sound, go even deeper into a state of relaxation." Because of the accompanying loud pings, immunizing against noise is also particularly helpful during MRI scans.

And use only the suggestions that are helpful for you.

Equally important as immunizing against noise is immunizing against unhelpful suggestions. When a patient hears suggestions while in trance, those suggestions can become powerfully embedded into the patient's subconscious. Unhelpful suggestions are always counterproductive to the procedure and can be harmful to the patient. A common misstep is choosing suggestions or imagery that although usually fine for most patients is unhelpful for the specific patient. For example, suggesting that the patient "visit" a meadow with beautiful flowers and scents would not be pleasant if the patient has pollen allergies. Briefly talking with the patient before beginning can help you avoid such pitfalls. Also, it is realistic to assume that while you are structuring hypnosis there will be other healthcare professionals who may feel a need to jump in to express their empathy. Unfortunately they may misguidedly choose negative suggestions and distractions.[1; 2]

> *"On one, you can do one thing—look up, on two, two things, slowly close your eyes and take a deep breath; and on three, three things, breath out, relax your eyes, and let your body float."*

The script uses a so-called "eye-roll" induction. Associating counts one, two, three with the number of steps needed for each count of the induction makes it easy to remember and repeat. After you introduce the eye roll with, *"There are a lot of ways to relax but here is one simple way,"* you can also say, "You can follow me along or first see how it works. It is a great way to relax yourself whenever you need and you can do this now or later or whenever you need to in the hospital or at home." Patients may follow your eye roll instructions right away. If they don't, you can say, "Looks pretty doable, hmm? What do you think?" Pause, and then repeat the instructions. You can also look up at the ceiling when you instruct the patient to *"look up."* You may even point to the ceiling with your hand. Also, take a deep breath in when instructing the patient to do so at sentence two, and breathe out audibly just after *"three things..."* or after completing the last sentence—making sure your patient doesn't need to keep their breath held too long. You may want to practice this.

> *Right now imagine that you are floating somewhere safe and comfortable, in a bath, a lake, a hot tub, or just floating in space, each breath deeper and easier. Just notice how with each breath you let a little more tension out of your body as you let your whole body float, safe and comfortable, each breath deeper and easier.*

You continue your induction with a paradox of floating through the table or—if a patient were in a chair—you can say, "floating right DOWN through the chair; emphasizing DOWN:

"That's good, just imagine your whole body floating down, floating through the table, with each breath deeper and easier."

This paradox contradicts the usual expectations of floating being directed upwards. The acceptance of such a statement becomes part of the hypnotic experience.[3] Hypnotic inductions can include suggestions for muscle relaxation, but they tend to be lengthy. Inducing a sensation of floating is the fastest way to relax the entire body.

Good. Now with your eyes closed and remaining in this state of concentration please describe for me how your body is feeling right now.

It is a good idea to check in early if there is resistance or if there is something that is stopping the patient from proceeding. Patients who are too anxious or too worried will not enter a hypnotic state. Therefore, at this early stage, we are asking the patient to tell us how his or her body is feeling. Note that patients can talk freely with you in hypnosis as compared to general anesthesia or heavy pharmacological sedation.

Where do you imagine yourself being; what is it like? Can you smell the air? Can you see what is around you?

If the patient expresses distress, you may need to proceed to the provisions for management of pain and distress in the script. Otherwise, you can continue with helping the patient structure his or her imagery by appealing to all of the senses. Some patients will tell you where they are; others want to keep it for themselves. It is okay either way.

Good. Now this is your safe and pleasant place to be and you can use it in a sense to play a trick on the doctors (or this whole procedure). Your body has to be here, but you don't. So just spend your time being somewhere you would rather be.

Once the patient has indicated verbally or by ideomotor signals that he or she is indeed in a good place, you can anchor the patient in this resourceful state. Ideomotor signals, which will be discussed in detail in chapter 15, "Ideomotor Signals," are nonverbal ways to communicate; such as requesting a nod of the head in agreement. Creating a safe space helps immunize against procedural reminders of old abuse and permits the patient to return to this safe space in case of abreactions—the violent reliving of past trauma.

You often find interspersed in the script: "Good." Slowly saying, "Good" or "mmhmm" with a pause, reassures the patient that things are going as expected. A "Good" or "mmhmmm" on and off may also be all you need to say during lengthy procedures to keep the patient in trance. These words not only reassure the people who hear them but also the person who says them out loud.

> *Now again with your eyes closed and remaining in the state of concentration, describe what you are feeling right now.*

Note the check-ins in the script of how the patient is feeling.

> *Now, if there is some discomfort, and there may be some with the procedure as they prepare you and insert the line, or as you feel the dye entering your body, there is no point in fighting it. You can admit it, but then transform that sensation. If you feel some discomfort, you might find it helpful to make that part of your body to feel warmer, as if you were in a bath. Or cooler, if that is more comfortable, as if you had ice or snow on that part of your body. This warmth and coolness becomes a protective filter between you and the pain. If you have any discomfort right now imagine that you are applying a hot pack or you are putting snow or ice on it and see what it feels like. Develop the sense of warm or cool tingling numbness to filter the hurt out of the pain. With each breath, breathe deeper and easier, your body is floating, filter the hurt out of the pain.*

The script contains suggestions in how to deal with pain and discomfort as a prophylactic measure and also to mitigate pain and discomfort once they are experienced. For procedures that include painful stimuli or extended uncomfortable positioning, it is helpful to set realistic expectations and not have patients feel they have failed if they experience discomfort. You cannot and should not promise that there will be no discomfort. Such a promise is not believable and may not be attainable. Instead, stick to the approach the script suggests. For example, Dr. Lang, right before and while applying the local anesthetic, sometimes says, "And you might experience some coolness, or numbness, or a delicious sensation of tingling."

You may notice that there are several more segments where the patient's feedback is requested. The actions to be followed depending on the response are self-explanatory in the script.

> *We are going to leave formally this state of concentration by counting backwards from three to one. On three get ready, on two with your eyes closed roll up your eyes, and on one let your eyes open and take a deep breath and let it out. That will be the end of the formal exercise, but when you come out of it you will still have the feeling of comfort that you felt during it. Ready, three, two, one. If necessary: Three—get ready. Two—with your eyes closed, roll up your eyes. One—let your eyes open and take a deep breath, and feel refreshed and proud about having helped yourself through this procedure.*

The conclusion of a hypnotic session is the reorientation to the waking state. Reorientation is another ritualized approach that can mirror the induction or use a different approach. Some hypnotists count up, others down for the transitions between trance and waking state. This is also the time when you can embed posthypnotic suggestions, which are suggestions the patient can carry beyond the session. We like adding the suggestion of feeling proud about having been able to help themselves though the procedure—this also acknowledges the patients' efforts in having learned this new skill. It also rounds up the initial premise of the script and procedure hypnosis in general: All you do is help patients help themselves. They do the real work and deserve all the credit.

Key Points to Remember

- You can successfully guide patients in self-hypnotic relaxation by reading a script.
- Sitting down with a script tends to comfort the patient, taking away notions of capricious power and hocus-pocus.
- Scripts facilitate learning the language of hypnosis.
- When working in teams, scripts help to foster a common language and facilitate the handing off of the patient—along with the script—among team members if the practitioner needs to leave the procedures room while the hypnosis is in progress.
- When building your own script include as minimum: an induction, immunization against noise and unhelpful suggestions, appropriate suggestions, anchoring in a safe place, and a reorientation to the waking state.

Opportunities to Practice

- Read again script 1.1, "Experiencing Confidence," to experience hypnosis yourself and also to identify the components of the script according to the examples and discussion presented in the analysis of the "Study Script" in this chapter.
- For now, hold off with practicing the script with patients until you have learned more of the techniques in the subsequent chapters.

CHAPTER 13
Inductions Using Eye Fixation or Movements

Case 13.1 The F—— Ceiling

Hemodialysis requires a way to take blood from the patient and return it after it has been cleaned by the kidney machine. A common solution is to create a dialysis fistula by joining a vein in the arm to one of the larger arteries so that rapidly flowing blood can be diverted up the vein. The vein enlarges and then can be easily punctured. Unfortunately narrowing in the blood vessels can develop and the blood going through the fistula clots repeatedly. Dr. Lang's team had just finished opening the clotted dialysis fistula of a young woman. The patient was visible through the lead glass windows of the procedure room; and Dr. Laser looked through the glass just as the patient started to develop a full-fledged allergic reaction to the contrast medium that had been used to visualize her blood vessels. The patient was screaming and writhing, wildly scratching herself all over, throwing herself around so that the doctors and nurses could barely keep her on the gurney. It was just a ghastly scene. A doctor administered some medication to stop the itch, but it didn't help. The team rolled the patient out of the procedure room into the holding area. The patient was yelling obscenities. Dr. Laser was asked to assist with calming the patient down.

Dr. Laser's offer to help was answered by "Get the hell out of there." Subsequent offers and suggestions were met by similar ribald rejections and suggestions—everything was fuck, suck, or whatever other expletive came to the patient's mind. Dr. Laser validated the patient and her dilemma by matching the patient's rhythm (See chapter 4, "Matching Rhythm to Lead") and part of the patient's language. Dr. Laser made several attempts to get the patient's attention and to elicit her cooperation to help her counteract the itching. At this point the patient was lashing out at anyone who approached her bed and refused to focus on what was being said to her. When Dr. Laser's usual measured approaches did not work, she firmly instructed the patient: "Okay, then just look at the fucking ceiling!" And after the stunned patient paused for a moment, Dr. Laser continued, "And your eyes won't close until your inner mind gives you permission." With that, Dr. Laser turned and walked away to give the patient space. Dr. Laser didn't look back knowing full well from her years of experience that getting the patient to focus her eyes upward and then to close them was the best chance to guide her into trance.

The surprised patient complied. She looked at the ceiling for a few moments, then closed her eyes and remained very quiet. The nurse who was with her came running after Dr. Laser. Dr. Laser found the patient in a deep trance and was able to guide the patient to immerse herself in a cool comfortable lake that would float away all the itching and soothe her skin.

Eventually, the patient was brought to the dialysis unit for a dialysis session. An hour later Dr. Lang's team received a call from the unit. The dialysis unit staff just could not figure out—and were very curious about—what had been done to the patient. They were amazed. They said they had never before seen the patient so cooperative. ***Case Notes, E. Laser***

What This Case Illustrates Suggesting that patients focus their eyes on an object until their eyes close helps patients enter trance.

Eye Movement Sequences for Trance Induction

To use hypnosis to help patients though procedures or medical tests, you need them to enter trance. *Trance* is the term used to describe an altered state of consciousness in which external realities become unimportant. You want patients to stop screening the environment and having unhelpful thoughts race through their mind. You want to calm their mind and induce a state of focus and relaxation. People can and do enter trance with the eyes open and defocused. Common examples of eyes-open trance include daydreaming and being absorbed in running, especially during a marathon. However, eye closure is helpful for medical encounters. Closed eyes keep out visual distractions. The strategy "out of sight, out of mind," is particularly helpful around syringes and other medical equipment and devices. In addition to keeping distractions out, eye closure can also be used as part of an induction—the ritualized invitation into hypnotic trance. You have already learned in chapter 12, "Hypnosis by Script," about the eye-roll induction, an upward gaze followed by closure and relaxation of the eye.

Many inductions are based on suggestions that invite the person to focus his or her eyes on a target—often but not always associated with an upward gaze—until the eyes fatigue and close.[1] The target can be a spot on the ceiling—ideally one of the patient's choosing—the back of the eyelids, a spot on the patient's forehead, any real or imagined feature in the surroundings, or commercial props. Despite the claims of the manufacturers, there is no evidence for the superiority of such devices.[2] Drs. Gail Gardner and Karen Olness describe eye fixation techniques with children. They have their young patients hold a coin, look at it until it falls down (to a place where it will be safe), and use the fall as signal for eye closure.[3]

One advantage of eye fixation or eye movement sequences is that they are straightforward and easy for patients to remember for subsequent use on their own. There is one caution: when you use eye fixation techniques, it is important to ask patients to relax their eyes at some point. This happens mostly automatically when patients close their eyes. Rarely a patient may keep the eyes strained in an upward or inward focused gaze after eye closure. More likely, you may have forgotten to instruct the eyes to relax during an eye roll induction. Evidence that the eyes are not relaxed is typically a jerky motion of the patient's eye muscles. If this occurs, just suggest that the patient, "relax all the tiny muscles in the eye and around the eye."

Relationship Between Eye Movements and Hypnotic Trance

There is scientific evidence of a connection between eye movements and hypnotic trance. Renowned psychiatrist and expert in hypnosis, Dr. Herbert Spiegel, (father of David Spiegel, author of the "Study Script", presented in chapter 12) stumbled on the association between vertical eye movements and trance when he noticed that one of his patients consistently looked up when going in trance.(4) Dr. Spiegel researched this phenomenon extensively and hypothesized that the neural circuitry that controls the upward gaze is genetically related to circuitry that controls imagination and focused attention. The consequence of this hypothesis is twofold: performing an eye roll should help a person's brain to get ready to enter trance; and a person who has great capacity to enter trance should also be good at performing an eye roll. Jun-Seok Lee at the Kwandong University, Gyunggi, Korea, and colleagues further supported this hypothesis on the interrelationship between eye roll and trance phenomena using modern fractal analysis of EEGs in the waking state and in hypnosis.(5)

They were able to show hypnosis-specific electrophysiological changes towards "white noise patterns" in the same areas of the brain that are also involved with the control of vertical eye movements, with planning for eye movements, with inhibition of eye movements, and with shifts of attention.

When guiding patients through an induction, you can sometimes see a tiny flutter of the closed eyelids. This is a cue that the patient is entering trance.

Observations of Eye Movements During Induction

When suggesting vertical eye movements for trance inductions, you may encounter the phenomenon of disappearing pupils.

JOURNAL ENTRY 13.1

Up to the Eyeballs

One of the newly trained residents read to a patient the "Study Script," using the induction with the vertical eye roll. When she instructed the patient to look up and then to slowly close his eyes, the patient's eye balls turned up, up, up, and up until there were only the white of the eyeballs seen—no more pupil in sight. The resident continued with reading the script but looked concerned. The patient entered a deep trance and the procedure started. The resident came to me somewhat distressed and explained that the white eyeballs really freaked her out. She thought the patient's eyes would get stuck in the forehead, and that she had gotten him into this situation. Would he be okay? She was quite relieved when I explained to her that not only was there no cause to worry, but that the white eyeballs were rather a sign that the patient was highly hypnotizable.

The case went well, and of course the pupils rolled back into place. The patient had a profound hypnotic experience, and was very pleased about this newly found ability to help himself because he had many more medical tests to go through. This success also greatly enhanced the resident's confidence and excitement about procedure hypnosis. ***Journal Notes, E Lang***

You may well experience patients whose eyes roll far up and back during eye roll inductions until only the whites of the eyes show. As mentioned in the journal entry above, the white eyeballs are evidence that the patient is highly hypnotizable. This conclusion is based on the Hypnotic Induction Profile test that Drs. Herbert and David Spiegel developed.[(6)] Their test grades the distance between the lower eyelid and the pupil on a scale of 0-4 with 4 indicating the highest hypnotizability and corresponding to a completely white eyeball.

Key Points to Remember

- Invitations for eye fixation and eye movements facilitate trance.
- Having patients close their eyes during induction keeps out visual distractions.
- When using eye fixation or eye roll inductions make sure to include subsequent suggestions to relax the eyes to avoid eyestrain.
- Areas in the brain that are involved in trance are also involved in eye movements, planning for eye movements, inhibition of eye movements, and shifts of attention.
- White eyeballs during upward gaze and eye closure are typically a sign of high hypnotic capacity and no cause for concern.
- A fine flutter of the closed relaxed eyelids is a cue that the patient is entering trance.

Opportunities to Practice

Set yourself up a sequence of eye roll (see Study Script 12.1) or other form of eye fixation with subsequent relaxation as a signal for you to enter a state of self-hypnosis and relaxation. Also develop a ritual for returning yourself to your natural state of awareness. You can use this induction for self-hypnosis when you want to take a quick refreshing break.

CHAPTER 14
Confusional Inductions

Case 14.1 The Mars Bar

During a training class with a radiology team, Dr. Lang passed out sample induction scripts prepared by Dr. Laser for the participants to use as they worked with one another to practice hypnosis. Many of the staff had never personally experienced hypnosis, and weren't sure about whether they would enter trance. The participants gathered into small groups and, in turn, read to one another the scripts. Some team members were able to easily enter trance. One of the technologists who very much wanted to experience hypnosis was not successful—she wanted hypnosis, but had a hard time letting go. This all changed when her group partner read the following induction script to her:

> You can go into a relaxed place at your own pace, you can relax deeply, and you can do this now, or in a moment from now. Everyone knows the importance of doing some homework. One never stops learning, so experience is a great teacher. There are lots of ways to get to a stoplight. When you first learn how to drive, while you think that it's important to stop, you might remember a time when you stepped on the gas to get there fast, and then you hurried up to stop.
>
> Now, your eyes won't close until your inner mind gives you permission. That's great, and it's nice to know that you might remember back sometime when you enjoyed sinking your teeth into a nice juicy peach, or into a nice Mars bar. That's right, and even though Mars has a bar, there are many bars in Mars. Did

you know that? Have you ever read about Mars, or maybe you saw it on Star Trek or Star Dreck. Yes, that's the ticket to go there now, or you may go to another place of interest that you might enjoy. A person can be resourceful in so many ways, and there are a variety of ways to solve a problem. While I don't know what you do, or enjoy doing, and I don't know what you like to do best, but it's a fun idea to explore and go to a place of fun, of pleasant surroundings, and peace.

Wow, let's be on our way. And while we are going there, the other part of you is here getting repaired to really enjoy everything possible. Time flies when we are having fun, and one can spend time in a variety of ways. You can focus on making the best use of time, while your playful self enjoys it. You don't even have to listen to my voice because your unconscious mind will hear it clearly. There is nothing you have to do right now, nothing you have to think about or respond to. You don't even have to expect anything in particular.

The participants had fun reading the script—a little humor goes a long way. The technologist who had been unable to enter trance with the other scripts, was very excited about having had a profound hypnotic experience with this one. She explained, "The Mars Bars really did it." ***Case Notes, E. Lang***

What This Case Illustrates When a person wants to go into trance but is experiencing resistance by staying consciously too vigilant, methods that confuse the conscious mind can help the person to let go and overcome resistance.

Overcoming Resistance to Induction

You may encounter patients who want to experience a state of hypnosis or relaxation but cannot let go right away. Sex may be an analogy. Some people get the full experience the first time they try, others may need longer or additional attempts before they trust themselves and the partner well enough to get there. For patients who want hypnosis but are unable to let themselves go into trance using the "Study Script," or other regular scripts, you can often help them by using a form of confusional induction, which include the confusion method and the conscious-unconscious dissociation method of induction.

The Confusion Method of Induction

Milton Erickson used the confusion method of induction with patients who either desperately wanted therapy but were too overwhelmed by their clinical problems and presuppositions to enter trance, or were—for known or unknown reasons—determined to show that hypnosis would not work on them.[1] Usually, the confusion method overcame such resistance.

Confusion type inductions use a conversational tone and confuse the mind by juxtapositions of seemingly contradictory and unrelated statements. The method may also rely on a play of words in which unobtrusively new ideas are inserted, such as in case 14.1, "The Mars Bar." With either approach, the patient's critical thinking can't keep up and tires while searching for a meaning. In this state of disorientation, people become more open to embedded suggestions.

Sometimes inserting an element of surprise or shock into the conversation achieves the goal.[2] Unexpected behavior on the part of the hypnotist may astonish the patient to such a degree that the patient becomes so at loss of what to do next that he or she will follow the next comprehensible suggestion made.[1] Case 13.1, "The F—— Ceiling," is an example of such an event. One can imagine the belligerent patient's surprise at Dr. Laser demanding unexpectedly, "Then just look at the fucking ceiling."

When you use the confusion method, you can proceed as you would usually do as soon as your patient enters trance.

And as usual, don't forget immunizations against noise and unhelpful suggestions. (See chapter 12, "Hypnosis by Script") You may use the following script to induce patients who want hypnosis but cannot stop themselves resisting it.

Script 14.1 Confusion Induction

You can go into a relaxed place at your own pace, you can relax deeply, and you can do this now, or in a moment from now.

Everyone knows the importance of doing some homework. One never stops learning, so experience is a great teacher.

There are lots of ways to get to a stoplight. When you first learn how to drive, while you think that it's important to stop, you might remember a time when you stepped on the gas to get there fast, and then you hurried up to stop.

Now, your eyes won't close until your inner mind gives you permission. Yes, that's right. And now, you can go down that bike path, riding down the trail, lowering down the hill, and you can go just as fast as your safety inner gauge allows you to go, and while the wind is blowing through your hair, and the sun is kissing your face, you can feel so free. And the constriction you might have felt, is leaving you, blowing in the breeze, and fading away in the air. And you know that that was a challenge, riding down that mountain, it is one thing to climb up, it's hard and it requires lots of work, and struggle, but all those past stifles, just enhanced your life up to now. And its good to know that while riding down this mountain, free as a bird, you can let go, yes let go, free of those past restrictions, that used to bind you and control you, so that now, while riding downhill on your bike, the limitless, unbound, open, released, feeling a new feeling of emancipation is wrapping you in a blanket of complete and utter energy. You no longer have to be chained and leashed to respond in the old ways, new and inviting behavior is taking charge. And you don't even have to listen to my voice, because you're unconscious mind will hear it clearly.

There is nothing you have to do right now, nothing you have to think about or respond to. You don't even have to expect anything in particular. And, time flies when we are having fun. And one can spend time in a variety of ways. You can focus on making the best use of time, while your playful self enjoys it. ***End of Script 14.1***

Conscious-Unconscious Dissociation Method of Induction

Another approach to confusional induction is to use conscious-unconscious dissociation suggestions. The idea is to link seemingly contradictory options that then leave the patient no alternative but to accept a desirable concept. As illustrated in "Script 14.2," when using conscious-unconscious dissociation suggestions, the statements flow in either of the following formats:

- "Your conscious mind _____(verb)_____ while *(alternately: and, or, since, as, at the same time)* your unconscious mind _____(verb)_____"
- "While your unconscious mind _____(verb)_____ your conscious mind _____(verb)_____."[2]

Script 14.2 Conscious-Unconscious Dissociation Induction

Your conscious mind might be listening to my voice while your unconscious mind is very busy attending to important matters; while your conscious mind may not fully trust hypnosis, your unconscious mind is concerned with what is safe; perhaps your conscious mind may be doubtful, but your unconscious mind can find security, because, it thinks in a broader scope; your conscious mind may be cautious and take precaution while your unconscious mind can often select the depth of trance it decides to go; and your conscious mind often knows and watches, while your unconscious mind protects and guides you; as your conscious mind may hear my words, while your unconscious mind can allow you to deepen your trance, and does hear and knows; while your conscious mind wonders how to, your unconscious mind already knows and discovers how.

End of Script 14.2

Key Points to Remember

- Confusional methods of induction are helpful for patients who want to experience hypnosis but are inhibited by their medical condition or feel they have to resist.
- Confusional methods tire critical thinking and permit the patient's subconscious mind to become open to suggestions.
- The confusion method of induction relies on an element of surprise and seemingly contradictory and unrelated statements with interspersed suggestions that facilitate trance.
- Conscious-unconscious dissociation links statements about the conscious and unconscious mind, which, even though that may seem contradictory, lead to the same desired outcome.

Opportunities to Practice

You may enjoy practicing conscious-unconscious mind double speak. You can start by making up 5 sentences of statements linking a conscious mind activity with an unconscious mind activity.

CHAPTER 15
Ideomotor Signals

Case 15.1 The Fingers Know

One year after providing training there, Dr. Lang visited a large free-standing MRI to film an educational video.[1] R——, one of the former trainees, is a registered nurse who specializes in helping patients through large core breast biopsies under MRI. In the video (which you can view at hypnalgesics.com), she demonstrates her approach, which flows like a natural conversation with the patient during the procedure.

To begin, a team of nurses and technologists place the patient on her belly on the procedure table. They prop the patient's chest up on pillows and position it over the biopsy contraption to provide access from the side to the breast. While the positioning is in progress, R—— places an IV in the patient's outstretched left hand. All the while the MRI machine is pinging like a fast, loud, gigantic metronome. R—— suggests that the patient allow the noises in the room to deepen her relaxation. R—— checks in with the patient, asking how she feels and if she is comfortable. The patient affirms this. After asking if it is okay to do so, R—— explains that she will touch the patient's back from time to time, and that when the patient feels her touch, the patient will go into even deeper relaxation. As R—— speaks, she anchors the patient using a firm touch on the patient's right back next to the shoulder. R—— continues, "When my voice is silent, I am still with you. And if you don't feel like speaking, you can signal me with your fingers." R—— goes on while carefully watching the patient's right hand, which is outstretched in front of the patient on R——'s side of the table. "You will know that one of your fingers is your Yes finger," says R——, "and one of your fingers is your No finger. And they will appear to you. And as you are relaxed, you will have the sensation that one finger wants to say yes. Do you happen to notice which finger is your Yes finger?" The patient lifts her right index finger. R—— replies "Okay, very good," while she continues taping the IV line to the table and proceeding in her nursing tasks. R—— asks, "And which finger is your No finger?" and the patients little finger lifts. "Okay, I understand that, excellent."

Later during the procedure, the room is darkened to reduce glare on the monitors in the adjacent control room, the MRI machine keeps pinging, and the physician gets ready to apply the local anesthetic. While R—— tears open a large package with the biopsy gun and the doctor draws up the lidocaine in a syringe, R—— says "Some of that numbing medicine is working in a few seconds now—as you breathe in and out, calm and relaxed." When the drilling noise of the biopsy apparatus is audible, R—— asks, "How are you doing? Are you okay?" and the Yes finger rises. R—— confirms and reassures with, "Good." There is no need to interrupt the patient's experience by requiring her to talk. ***Case Notes, E. Lang***

What This Case Illustrates Finger movements can be used to communicate simple statements during medical procedures. This form of body language provides quick, honest answers, presumably right from the subconscious mind. Suggesting that patients use finger movement signals obviates the need of verbal answers, which can interrupt the patient's state of focused concentrations and are more prone to editing and censoring by the conscious mind.

Involuntary Motor Signals

Ideomotor refers to a subconscious idea being expressed as an involuntary or automatic motor signal.[2] For example, a person may nod in agreement without being fully aware of this behavior, or may shake the head while saying yes. A person's body language may be in agreement with what the person says or may contradict it. Milton Erickson liked to elicit ideomotor signaling in the form of non-voluntary nodding or shaking of the head in response to questions to get at real answers.[3] The psychologist Leslie LeCron together with obstetrician-gynecologist David Cheek built on Erickson's work and expanded on the use of ideomotor signaling. They experimented with Chevreul's Pendulum to demonstrate that the subconscious can produce physical movements beyond the control of the conscious mind. Chevreul's Pendulum refers to the work of Michel-Eugene Chevreul, a French natural scientist who in the 1830s conducted research with a pendulum suspended from a subject's finger to discover what powered the change in the direction of the pendulum's swing. LeCron and Cheek used a similar pendulum that swings in different directions in response to very slight—often imperceptible—movements of the person holding it.[4-6] The classic approach for using Cheveul's Pendulum is to draw a circle with a cross inside it and ask the subject to hold the pendulum, suspended from a finger, over the image. The subject is asked to decide which direction of pendulum motion—up and down, side-to-side, diagonal, clockwise or counterclockwise represent "yes," "no," and sometimes other designations as well. LeCron and Cheek instructed patients to use the pendulum to indicate "yes," "no," "I am not ready to answer the question consciously yet," and "I don't know." LeCron and Cheek found that the pendulum method was capable of signaling subconscious answers that could subsequently be brought to the patient's awareness and used to help solve therapeutic puzzles. The pendulum proved an effective tool for discovering subconscious information, but its physical and positional requirements limit its use. Consequently, hypnotists used fingers for ideomotor signaling for greater ease of use and adaptability to all situations.

During patient sedation without medication, ideomotor signals come in handy when one wishes to get answers without requiring the patient to talk. Ideomotor finger movements can be used with patients in hypnosis or in a waking state. Identification of a Yes finger and a No finger are quite sufficient for this purpose, although adding an I Don't Know Yet finger may sometimes be useful. The finger responses can be used to obtain feedback on questions of comfort as in case 15.1 "The Fingers Know." Ideomotor signals also makes it easier for patients to indicate when they are not comfortable. Patients sometimes hold back from verbally expressing what they need for fear of not hurting the feelings of the hypnotist or medical team. Ideomotor signals also help the practitioner stay on track during hypnosis by providing easy and honest patient feedback about execution of suggestions or choice of imagery.

Establishing Ideomotor Signals

Surgeon Dabney Ewin uses hypnosis both preoperatively and postoperatively as part of his care of patients who must undergo surgery. To gain access to the patient's subconscious mind to identify fears, past experiences, expectations, misconceptions, etc., he employs ideomotor signals. For positioning the patient to aid execution and observation of ideomotor signals, Dr. Ewin suggests keeping the patient's wrist flexed.[(2)] The flexed position—palm moved toward the front of the forearm—keeps the extensor muscles of the arm tight, ensuring that the slightest muscular contraction will produce a visible movement of the finger. This positioning may not be feasible in every case or throughout some cases, but its benefit warrants making an effort to use it when possible. During procedures or medical tests, it is best to focus on the patient's hand that is closest to you and/or is not covered by drapes or limited in its ability to move. To program the fingers for signaling, you can use verbiage similar to that used by R—— in case 15.1, "The Fingers Know," or ask the patient's subconscious mind to select any one of the fingers as the Yes finger. Explain that the patient can lift the chosen finger to "say" yes. When the Yes finger is identified, then ask that the No finger be lifted. If the person cannot identify the fingers right away, give him or her a little time. Ask the patient if one of his or her fingers feels different then the other fingers. Say that the finger may feel heavy or it might wiggle or tingle or lift on its own or feel weird; explain that the finger that is different in such a way is the Yes finger. Repeat the same explanation for the No finger. The movements of the fingers can be very subtle. You must watch carefully for the slightest movement. Optionally, you can reinforce the assignment of the finger by stroking it gently and lifting it to give sensory feedback to the patient.

Ideomotor Signals for Exploration of Thought

You may occasionally wonder about your own motivations or doubts. Checking in with oneself by using ideomotor signaling can be revealing. Your subconscious mind may surprise you. This is true of anyone. Perhaps you are asked from time to time by friends or colleagues for personal advice. As the Journal Entry that follows illustrates, often the best answers to personal problems are those revealed through ideomotor signals from one's own fingers.

JOURNAL ENTRY 15.1

Decisions, Decisions

S—— had just returned from a one-month visit to a prestigious institution in a different city. S—— had loved the intellectual simulation, the international flair of the place, the buzz, and the opportunity to branch out into new fields of interest. S—— had done a great job there, too, and was offered a position; albeit at a considerably lower salary than S——'s present one. S—— had worked at the current institution for many years, was well established, and familiar with—although sometimes put off by—the local politics. The necessary relocation that came with accepting the job offer, by chance, provided an easy way out of a long-term relationship that had come to a state of staleness and occasional irritation. On top of it all S——'s mother, who lived thousands of miles away, had started to insist on S——'s moving back home to help in the fledgling family business the parents had launched. Unfortunately, in the family business location, there would have been very limited opportunities for S—— to pursue the newly found professional dreams and interests. S—— was stressed with the options: stay in the current job and relationship, move to help the parents, accept new job offer and move there. S—— could not decide and came to me to discuss this personal dilemma.

While I could suggest points to consider S—— might not have thought of, I have learned over the years that one really cannot advise other people on their relationships and passions. One simply never has all the facts of people's inner workings. I have also learned over the years that deep own in one's gut, one does know where things stand, even if one does not want to admit it openly. I told S—— that I would support whatever the decision would be and do what I could to make it work. With regard to the decision itself, my suggestion was for S—— to identify a Yes finger and a No finger and an I Don't Know Yet finger and to use those identified fingers to access S——'s own deeper knowledge of the situation and to reveal that knowledge to the conscious mind. S—— was surprised to see these fingers identify themselves so quickly. I suggested that S—— ask the fingers the same questions S—— had for me—and to do so privately to see what the subconscious answers would be. S—— could then take those answers as a guide. S—— felt quite empowered by this approach and left in better spirits.

A few months later S—— called me. S—— had reached decisions and acted on them. S—— was quite happy having realized what really mattered and with the course life had taken. S—— felt that although it was tough going, that the direction was the right one leading towards fulfillment of previously hidden passions and aspirations. ***Journal Notes, E. Lang***

Key Points to Remember

- Ideomotor signals are a form of body language that provides quick honest answers presumably right from the subconscious mind.
- Ideomotor signals come in handy when one wishes to get answers without making the patient talk.
- You can use ideomotor finger signals in the waking state and in hypnosis.
- Identification of a Yes and a No finger are quite sufficient, although adding an I Don't Know Yet finger may sometimes be useful.
- A flexed wrist position makes it easier to see which fingers are moving—but is not obligatory.
- Ideomotor signals can be helpful when you wish to explore your own motivations or gain insight from your subconscious mind.

Opportunities to Practice

- Take a moment of quiet and sit down. With your hand relaxed in your lap, ask yourself which finger is the Yes finger? The No finger? The I Don't Know Yet finger? If the fingers don't reveal themselves right away, you can test with repeated questions for which you know the answers such as "Is today the 4th of July?" "Is my car green?"
- If you have a question about your motives or an upcoming decision, use your ideomotor signals. You may be surprised at the answers.

CHAPTER 16

Uses and Misuses of *Trying*

Case 16.1 Trying is Not Doing

A visitor to the radiology department overheard a conversation between a patient waiting outside the procedure suite and the nurse who was going to assist the patient through his interventional radiology procedure. The patient was in significant pain and was concerned that lying on the procedure table for an extended time would make his pain worse. He expressed his concern to the nurse, who assured him that she would take care of him during the procedure and would be "trying to make him comfortable throughout the whole procedure." The word *trying* stuck in the visitor's mind. With the patient out of sight, the visitor asked Dr. Lang, "What did '*trying* to make him comfortable' mean? Are there problems? Is the patient so badly off that he can't be helped? Or don't they know what they are doing here? If the nurse isn't sure that she knows how to help the patient be comfortable during this procedure, isn't there someone else here who does?" ***Case Notes, E. Lang***

What This Case Illustrates People often use the word *trying* to indicate that they are making a sincere effort to achieve something. The term, however, inherently carries the possibility of failure. *Trying*, even at its most earnest, promises attempting but offers no guarantee of succeeding. It is this presupposition of the possibility of failure that triggers feelings of doubt and can cause stress in people being told that someone is "trying" rather than "doing."

Ambiguity of Trying

Try is an ambiguous word that can convey several meanings—sometimes unintentionally. Try is casually and commonly used to indicate an attempt at getting something done. The speaker's spoken message, as in case 16.1, "Trying is Not Doing," is "I'm trying." The speaker may be hoping to communicate: I'm attempting to get this done; I'm doing my best; I couldn't do more. However, most people are aware, at least subconsciously, that a person's use of the word *try* signals his or her acceptance of the possibility that he or she will not come through. Therefore, when a speaker says, "trying," the listener may also hear the unspoken background message: "Other people or events or circumstances out of my control may keep me from succeeding."

If you are unsure of your sensitivity to the implied prospect of failure in *trying*, consider how often you hear the word used in the past tense as a prologue to statements of failure. For example, when a speaker begins, "I tried really hard to pass this exam—or finish the project, or get the job, etc.," do you automatically expect to hear the speaker next say, "but I flunked, couldn't do it, or didn't get it?" Beginning a statement with "I tried," doesn't necessarily signal lack of success, of course, but when it does, the statement usually includes a valid reason for the failure—other people, events, or circumstances out of the speaker's control sabotaged success. On the other hand, if a speaker instead begins, "I worked really hard to pass this exam, or etc.," are you equally suspicious that he or she is about to announce failure? Probably not; of course, "I worked really hard on ...," can precede, "but I just couldn't ...," nevertheless, the possibility is not so expected. The point is that *try* alerts the listener upfront to an uncertain outcome. Not using *try* doesn't guarantee success, it just eliminates your admission that you might fail or have failed.

Developing and maintaining the patient's trust in the medical team and nurturing the patient's expectations that things will go well are important. Being unaware of a language habit of using *try* when indicating desire to *do* can undermine the patient's trust in the caretakers' abilities, and shake the patient's optimistic outlook. If you want to indicate your efforts, other options include: "I will give my very best to...," "I am working on ...," "I will keep at ...," "I will use all the tricks known to medicine to ..." or best of all, when you can reasonably assume you can, simply say, "I will ...."

Equally important is using words other than *try* when inviting patients to do things you actually want them to do. Instead of saying, "Would you like to try some hypnosis?" you can say, "Would you like to experience hypnosis?" The second statement expresses your trust in the person to follow though. "Please try to get up onto this table," gives the message that you have doubts about the patient's agility. If instead, you just say, "Please come up on the table," you leave all options open. You will find out soon enough if the patient needs more help to do so. Often just leaving *try* out of your sentence will suffice.

Uses of *Trying* in Hypnosis

Interestingly, there are times in hypnosis when you want the patient to NOT succeed in following your suggestion. In such cases, using the word *try* works very well in making sure the patient doesn't "do." For example, if you instruct patients to try as hard as they can to keep their eyes open, they will invariably close them after a while. Or, if you want to demonstrate to patients that they are so relaxed that they either cannot or do not want to open their eyes; you can invite them to "try" to open their eyes. This exchange of your suggesting that they try to open their eyes, and their eyes remaining closed, helps patients notice that this in-hypnosis state of mind is different from the usual waking state. This suggestion to try to open the eyes when you know the patient's eyes will remain closed can serve as trance ratification.

Milton Erickson used the term *trance ratification* to describe the practice of providing patients with physical evidence that they have been hypnotized or that they can experience hypnotic effects.[1] For example, the practitioner may suggest to the patient in hypnosis that he or she experience a feeling of buoyancy in one arm, as if the arm is being pulled up by a big balloon, and the arm lifts and remains in a lifted position. When the patient is then re-alerted to the waking state and sees his or her arm still effortless up in the air, the patient may wonder how the arm got there and accepts the upheld arm as physical evidence that something unusual has happened. This confirmation of having been in a trance state demonstrates to the patient the power of his or her subconscious mind, and can, thus, instill hope, belief, and positive expectancy for hypnosis.[2] Once you have demonstrated to a patient that he or she is capable of trance, the patient becomes more willing and interested in following further suggestions or possibly entering deeper levels of trance. We find this to be the case with script 16.1, "The Floating Stone," which uses the term try several times in this context. We use this script for lengthy interventions, when we expect more intense procedure stimuli, and/or when we prefer patients to enter a deep trance.

Script 16.1 The Floating Stone

Become loose and comfortable; comfort is the key. It's just like you and I going on a brief vacation. You may hear outside noises, but they will only help you to deepen your own experience. And use only the suggestions that are helpful for you.

You can begin by looking up at a spot on the ceiling, high above your forehead. That's right. You may notice how your eyes begin to relax, and feel very heavy. There are very tiny little eyelid muscles in your eyelids, and they are very easy to control. Relax them completely to a point where they will not work. And when you are sure, and be sure in your own mind, and you have made the decision that they are completely relaxed to a point where they will not work, it is important to test and try to see that they will not work. Try now to open your eyes—but why bother. Okay, now stop trying.

Now you can send that relaxed feeling that you have in your eyelids throughout your entire face, your neck, feeling your jaw relaxing; your lips separating; and even your hair relaxing, too. Now allow this relaxation to spread throughout your whole body, from the top of your head to the tip of your toes.

Now, you can allow yourself to see the healing color of purple and all its glorious hues, or the color of your choice. And you can dive into this color, into all its delicious tones and shimmering lights, and feel wrapping all its gorgeous hues around you in a blanket of anesthesia and bliss, allowing your body to feel relaxed, calm, numb, courageous, and safe. You may feel numb just where it needs to be numb and for as long as it needs to be so. Relaxed, calm, numb, courageous, and safe. And this will be your mantra from now on as you begin to inhale. Breathe in to the count of four through your nostrils, pause into the gap, and exhale down through your nostrils all the way down and out to the count of eight. And continue this breathing through the entire time. In to the count of four, pause, and exhale through your nostrils all the way down and out continuing to say your words, your mantra: *relaxed, calm, numb, courageous, and safe.*

So now, we can begin to descend even deeper still. Go to a pleasant place, a beautiful safe place. A place of comfort and tranquility, a place of your choice. It might be on a mountain top with a creek, or home in your bed, or on a beach somewhere, or floating in the water of a lake or a pool, or even walking down a path. Wherever you find yourself, you can go there now, and you can begin to go down three deeper floors of hypnosis. And you can do this with your imagination and your imagination alone.

Perhaps you might enjoy seeing someone on the shore skipping a stone on the surface of the calm clear lake. As the stone ripples along, all worries and negative feelings that are not helpful to you ripple away. Then the stone comes to a place where it begins to float down. As you imagine the stone floating down to reach floor *A* you are floating to floor *A* of trance. And just as the stone freely floats down further, you descend along in your mind gently and safely to your floor *B* of trance. That's right. And when you are at floor *B* you can try to formulate the letter *B* but it is not possible. You cannot, no matter how hard you try, say the letter *B*. Try now. That's right. And as the stone begins to float down even further still, all the way down to the deepest level *C*, so can you allow yourself in your mind to go along down all the way to floor *C* of trance. Once again you can try to say, "*C*", but no matter how hard you try, you cannot say the letter *C*. You can also try to pick up your leg *(or lift your hand or thumb or whatever—depending on the procedure),* but you cannot. No matter how hard you try, you cannot raise your leg *(or lift your hand, etc.).* This is a very deep level.

And, as you allow yourself to continue your breathing, in to the count of four, pause, into the gap, and exhale through your nostrils to the count of eight, down and out, you continue to repeat your words: *relaxed, calm, numb, courageous, and safe.*

And now, when you are ready to ascend again to your natural sate of awareness, you can float up from floor *C* to *B* and then to *A*. You can take with you the memory of only the pleasant things about this experience and the pride of knowing how you can help yourself so well. You can take this positive and pleasant feeling with you. You can count from one to five and with each count becoming more alert, more refreshed. One: getting ready. Two: starting to open your eyes. Three: gently stretching. Four: further opening your eyes. And five: being fully alert, refreshed, delighted, and proud of how you have been able help yourself through this procedure. ***End of Script 16.1***

Key Points to Remember

- Most people are aware, at least subconsciously, that a person's use of the word try signals his or her acceptance of the possibility that he or she will fail.
- Making a language habit of using *try,* when wanting to indicate effort, can undermine the patient's trust in the caretakers' abilities and shake a patient's optimistic outlook.
- Omit *try* if you want to indicate efforts to achieve something. Just omit the word.
- Omit *try* when you invite patients to do something you want them to do.
- There are times in hypnosis when you want the patient to NOT be able to do something. Just use try while suggesting the activity you do not want to occur.
- This suggestion to try to do something (such as open their eyes) when you know the patients will not follow the suggestion (e.g. the eyes will remain closed) can serve as trance ratification, a demonstration to a patient the power of his or her subconscious mind.

Opportunities to Practice

- Describe for yourself your past achievements and the effort it involved to obtain them. Note what words you use to describe the effort and outcome. Did you use *try* in this context?
- Notice when you say *try.* Do you use it in situations where you believe you can succeed? If so, how do your patients or communication partners react to it? Is there a difference in their reaction when you use other words such as "I will ..." or "I am doing ..."

- Listen for the word *try* when people talk. When do people tend to use it most? If they use it in the past or present tense, do they follow with a "but…" disclaimer? How do they use it for future statements?
- Pick a spot in your field of view and try to keep your eyes open. Keep telling yourself "I am really trying hard to keep my eyes open." How long can you keep trying?

CHAPTER 17

Direct and Indirect Language

Case 17.1 You Are So Relaaaxed

Two publishers, in relatively short sequence, each sent Dr. Lang a hypnosis tape for review. The first tape used direct command-like suggestions and made clear predictions of what the listener was to experience. The listener was told—more than once—that he or she was to feel so relaaaxed. Then the tape listed in detail exactly what the listener was to do and what he or she should feel. The more Dr. Lang listened to the instructions and the predictions that she would experience first this and then that, the more her inner rebel said, "The heck I will." and "Don't bet that this will happen." Listening to the direct suggestions tape turned out to be a very long 40 minutes; during none of which was she very relaaaxed.

In contrast, the tape from the other publisher was structured around open suggestions. The listener was invited to imagine a space and decorate it as desired. Many options were offered at every step of the tape and the listener could choose those that seemed to fit the occasion and/or the listener's preferences. With this tape, Dr. Lang actually did feel very relaxed. Dr. Lang enjoyed her trance, and although this tape was slightly longer than the first one, the time she spent listening to this open-suggestion tape seemed to go by much quicker than did her review of the direct-commands one. ***Case Notes, E. Lang***

What This Case Illustrates People usually don't like to be told what to do. Direct, command-like suggestions can build resistance, but when indirect language and permissive suggestions are part of the offering, people tend to follow.

Direct Versus Indirect Suggestions

When you convey information to or make requests of patients or colleagues, you can do so in either an authoritarian, direct or indirect, permissive manner. Compare the following statements:

- **Direct:** Look at the ceiling.
- **Indirect:** You may want to look at a spot on the ceiling; any one you like.
- **Direct:** Your eyes feel relaxed.
- **Indirect:** You might be surprised to find the small muscles in your eyes relaxing.
- **Direct:** Help me out here, please.
- **Indirect:** I wonder if you could help me for a moment?

Milton Erickson was renowned for using indirect, permissive suggestions in what is sometimes called "Ericksonian" language, but he also used direct, authoritarian suggestions with some patients if indicated by their preference.[1] There is debate in hypnosis circles about which approach yields superior results.[2]

These approaches are clearly different, but one is not superior to the other. As Erickson found, there really is no one-size-fits-all approach; rather, the best choice is dependent on the situation at hand. One factor is individual personal preferences. Some patients seem to, in general, respond better to one approach or the other. Preferences, however, can change with circumstances. In our experience, for most people in the beginning of procedure hypnosis and in elective medical settings, indirect suggestions seem the best choice. On the other hand, patients in emergency states or already in trance seem to respond best to direct suggestions. Routinely, you may want to begin induction with indirect suggestions, and then smoothly segue into more direct suggestions once the patient is in trance or when you need to address an acute medical problem. For example, in patients who are in panic from an asthma attack or allergic reaction, Dr. Lang sometimes authoritatively tells the patients, "Breath in...and breath out... breath in...and out..., and breath in...and out...in...and out..., etc.," until the patient's acute state is broken and he or she can follow other suggestions or until medications can be given.

Once you start using indirect permissive language, using it can become second nature. Dr. Lang often catches herself starting her e-mails with requests, "I wonder if you might be able to help me with ...." In nonemergency situations, most people prefer to be asked permissively; not ordered.

Indirect Suggestions

To make indirect suggestions, use words such as *allow, can, may,* and *might.* Phrases that frame indirect suggestions include the following: *I wonder if you noticed..., You may notice changes within..., As you notice..., You may want to..., If possible..., If you are willing..., You could..., or It's fine to wait to see how you feel....*

When there is a particular outcome that you would like to help the patient experience, you might use *contingent suggestions,* which are two part statements that connect an observable or ongoing behavior or inevitable event with the outcome you want to help the patient experience. The basic templates for contingent suggestions are: As you do *X,* you may notice *Y,* and You won't do *X,* until *Y.*[2] You can also link several contingent suggestions together, and when appropriate, offer the patient choices. As you read through the following sample of induction dialogue, you may want to note the indirect suggestions integrated into the sentences and identify the contingent suggestions:

> Your eyes won't close until your inner mind gives you permission. As you are lying here, you might feel a little tingling and you might find one part of your body feeling different. As you are continuing to listen to my voice, I've noticed that your breathing has slowed a bit, and down you can float, letting go. You feel like you might be floating on a cloud or on a magic carpet, flying over a place you might like to visit again or that you have always wanted to visit. And now... *(validate what you see, responding to the patient in reference to what you notice, such as "that you are breathing more slowly," or "have your hand relaxed against your side,")* and as you travel to your destination, you may be experiencing some numbness in your hand or somewhere in your body and that's all right, and your eyes might want to close down and seal shut. You can develop numbness in your hand as you drop it into ice cold water, and you can move it to another place and transfer the numbness to your face and your tooth, but that tooth can stay in trance even though you can sink into the bed, dreaming of a ride on a bus to a beautiful place. Yes, that's good. I don't know where you are, but I have noticed that you might be going deep down into a deep relaxed place, and that's all right. You can go into your unconscious mind...go there now, and into the most wonderful opportunity to heal, have fun, and mend. There is no use waiting any longer. It is there now, so you can go way down, deeper and deeper, into the most relaxed feeling you ever had. There's no sense in holding you back. Things occur in their own way and time. As you allow yourself to reach your goal, it's important to slide down into trance and go inside yourself. You can go into a relaxed place at your own pace. You can relax deeply, and you can do this now, or in a moment from now.

Comparison of Scripts Featuring Either Direct Suggestions or Indirect Suggestions

To further illustrate the contrast between a script based on direct suggestions and a script based on indirect suggestions, we have created two somewhat extreme example scripts. These examples, as much as possible, each adhere to a single approach. As you read through each script, you might want to notice the language that most characterizes its approach.

Script 17.1 Progressive Muscle Relaxation: Direct Suggestions Approach

Allow your body to relax and rest comfortably against the table and get ready to close your eyes. Now slowly take a breath in through your nose...hold it...then exhale out through your mouth. Once again, take a deep breath in through your nose... hold it...then exhale through your mouth. That's right. Slowly taking a deep breath in through your nose, and out through your mouth, and continue focusing on the sound of my voice, and allow yourself to relax completely, feeling calm and comfortable and fully at ease.

Now I would like to do an exercise with you to show your body the difference between tension and relaxation, focusing on some of the smallest muscles in your body; the muscles in your eyes. I would like you to continue focusing on your breathing: in through your nose, out through your mouth. And now I would like to invite you to focus on the muscles in your eyes. Tense those muscles as hard as you can. Really allow them to become tight and hard. That's right, really tense. Tighten your eye muscles.

In a moment, I am going to count to three, and when I get to three, you will be able to release all the tension in your eyes, allowing them to become fully relaxed and at ease. One...really feel the tension...Two...tight, tight, tight...Three...now, allow your eye muscles to become completely relaxed and limp. Good.

Now, notice the sensation of this relaxing feeling. Allow this relaxing sensation to flow from your eyes, up into your eyebrows, and now up over the top of your head. Continue breathing deeply, and with each breath, allow the relaxation to spread...over the top of your head, now down the back of your head, over your ears, and down into your neck. Let this pleasant and soothing sensation now cause your whole head and neck to become completely relaxed and at ease.

With each breath you inhale, you inhale relaxation. And with each breath you exhale, you exhale any tension and any discomfort, any stress and whatever else you may want to let go of. Good.

Now, inhaling calming relaxation, and exhaling as you cleanse your body of tension. Almost as if you breathe the tension right out of your body through the pores of your skin.

Now, allow the sensation to spread down your shoulders... down your arms and your hands, and right down to the tips of your fingers. Let the relaxation spread across your back, and down through your abdomen...into your legs, and down through your calves, to the tips of your toes. Good.

And now, to show how successful you are at relaxing, I'd like to ask you if there's any place in your body that would like to feel even more relaxed than it already is *(wait for response, then continue.)* So take a very deep breath...hold this breath... now exhale. This is called a *signal breath.* It is your way of signaling your body to allow yourself to become even more fully relaxed and comfortable. When you take your signal breath, imagine that you are inhaling relaxation and comfort, and allow that breath to focus on the very spot of your body that you would like to feel even more relaxed. Now inhale relaxation, and allow the exhaled breath to go right to that spot, and breath any tension right out through the skin at that spot. Let the relaxation and calm replace any feeling of tightness, discomfort, or tension.

Now anytime during the procedure that you would like to feel more relaxed and more comfortable, you will be able to remember to use your signal breath to breathe calming relaxation to that spot to help you feel completely at ease.

You will notice lots of noises around you during the procedure; people will be talking and moving, the equipment will make noises, and the lights will go on and off quite often. As you are aware of these things, you will be able to allow them to take you even deeper into a state of complete relaxation and comfort.

While the procedure is under way, you may have questions about what's going on around you. You know that you can remain in your fully relaxed state of calm, and still be able to ask whatever questions you would like. I will answer them for you, or I will find out the answers for you.

When the procedure is completed, or whenever you decide, you can return to your regular alert state by simply counting from one to three, either in your head or out loud. When you do this, you will find that even in your alert and fully attentive state you will continue to benefit from the calming sense of relaxation you now feel. And you can return to this place of calm whenever you like, by simply closing your eyes for a moment, counting back from three to one, and taking your signal breath. ***End of Script 17.1***

Script 17.2 Progressive Muscle Relaxation: Indirect Permissive Suggestions Approach

I would like to invite you to begin—either with your eyes open or closed—by allowing your body to relax and rest comfortably against the table. Now you may want to slowly take a breath in through your nose...hold...then exhale out through your mouth. At your own pace, you can take again a deep breath in through your nose...hold it...then exhale through your mouth.

Now, as you continue this deep, relaxing breathing, you may be surprised to notice how just the act of breathing alone can help your body to relax and feel more comfortable. You might be curious to find out how you can relax your body even more. You can do this by focusing on some of the smallest muscles in your body: the muscles in your eyes. You may tighten those muscles as hard and close the eyes as firmly as you can. You will know when these muscles are as tight as they can be, and then you can you enjoy the wonderful feeling of letting their tension go, having them become completely relaxed and limp. Or you may not even need to tighten them first, and can just send a delicious sensation of relaxation down into these tiny muscles. And the muscle of your right eye may relax first or the muscle of your left eye may relax fist, or both may relax together; or they already may be so relaxed that they wouldn't work even if you tried.

You might experience this feeling of relaxation as pleasant warmth, or you might see a calming white light. Now you can allow this relaxing sensation to flow from your eyes, up into your eyebrows, and now up over the top of your head. And while you continue to breathe deeply and naturally, you may notice how with each breath the relaxation spreads...over the top of your head, down the back of your head, over your ears, and down into your neck. You can let this pleasant and soothing sensation now cause your whole head and neck to become completely relaxed and at ease.

And you may focus now on your breath; with each breath you inhale, you inhale relaxation. And you will notice how with each breath you exhale, you exhale any tension and any discomfort and any stress that you might be feeling. Good. It is almost as if you can breath the tension right out of your body through the pores of your skin.

Now, you may allow the sensation to spread down your shoulders...down your arms and your hands, and right down to the tips of your fingers. You might enjoy feeling how the relaxation spreads across your back, and down through your abdomen...into your legs, and down through your calves, to the tips of your toes. That's right. And if there's any place in your body that would like to feel even more relaxed than it already is you can notice its location without forcing or willing it. You can just take a very deep breath...hold this breath...and now exhale. This is called a *signal breath.* It can become your way of signaling your body to allow yourself to become even more fully relaxed and comfortable. When you take your signal breath, you can imagine that you are inhaling relaxation and comfort, and allow that breath to focus on the very spot of your body that you would like to feel even more relaxed. And now or in a few moments you can use your signal breath and inhale relaxation, and allow the exhaled breath to go right to that spot, and breathe any tension right out through the skin at that spot. You know when you will be ready to let relaxation and calm replace any feeling of tightness, discomfort, or tension; it may be now or in a few moments from now.

Now any time during the procedure that you would like to feel more relaxed and more comfortable, you can use your signal breath to breathe calming relaxation to that spot to help you feel completely at ease.

You may notice lots of noises around you during the procedure; people will be talking and moving, the equipment will make noises, and the lights will go on and off quite often. As you are aware of these things, just allow them to take you even deeper into a state of complete relaxation and comfort.

While the procedure is under way, you may have questions about what's going on around you. You know that you can remain in your fully relaxed state of calm, and still be able to ask whatever questions you would like. I will answer them for you, or I will find out the answers for you.

When the procedure is completed, or whenever you decide, you can return to your regular alert state by simply counting from one to three, either in your head or out loud. When you do this, you will find that even in your alert and fully attentive state you will continue to benefit from the calming sense of relaxation you now feel. And you can return to this place of calm whenever you like, by simply closing your eyes for a moment, counting back from three to one, and taking your signal breath. ***End of Script 17.2***

The above scripts are not typical. It would be unusual to use only direct or only indirect suggestions in the same session or script. In a real-life situation, you can adapt the style based on the patient's reaction. However, you can also compare the effect each approach has on you and what you might prefer. Perhaps one of the above single approach scripts plainly appealed more to you than the other. You may want to keep in mind, though, that this preference can also be affected by the state of mind and situation a person finds him- or herself in at any given moment, and that there are times when you may respond better to the one approach or the other.

To create the single-approach script examples, we adapted a progressive muscle relaxation script Dr. Lang's group had used prior to the institution of the "Study Script,"12.1. The original version of the Progressive Muscle Relaxation script, which contains both direct and indirect suggestions, appears in the "Script Appendix." You may notice how long this type of induction is. You can use progressive muscle relaxation when you have lots of time or when a patient does not want to "go anywhere," and just wants "to relax."

Key Points to Remember

- Indirect, permissive suggestions help reduce resistance.
- There really is no one-size-fits-all approach to language; rather the best choice—direct or indirect—is always dependent on the situation at hand.

- At the beginning of procedure hypnosis and in elective medical settings, indirect suggestions seem the best choice for most people.
- Patients in emergency states and when in trance respond best to direct suggestions.
- Contingent suggestions are two-part statements that connect an observable or ongoing behavior or inevitable event with the outcome you want to help the patient experience.
- It would be unusual to use only direct or only indirect language in the same session or script.
- Progressive muscle relaxation is suitable when you have lots of time or when a patient does not want to "go anywhere," and just wants "to relax."

Opportunities to Practice

- Read the above direct and indirect scripts aloud and reflect on your reaction afterwards. Did they get you in a hypnotic mood? Do you have a preference?
- Notice the kind of language—direct or indirect—that you use during your daily practice.
- If your work includes instructing patients for the same task many times a day, compare how direct and indirect suggestions affect patient's willingness and speed to follow through; for example, "Please lie down with your head up here and feet down there," verses "I wonder if you might now lie down with your head up here and your feet there." You may develop a sense for what phrasing may work best for which type of patient and/or situation.

CHAPTER 18
Imagery

Case 18.1 The Lady in the Red Dress

To acquire images using MRI technology, patients are surrounded by the powerful magnetic field that the MRI scanner creates; and they must hold still for 20 to 50 minutes, depending on the body part being scanned. Traditionally, the patient is positioned on a table and then the table is slid into the tubelike magnet scanner that produces the field. Many people have difficulty coping with the confined space. "Open" magnets, which do not encircle the entire patient, help deal with this sense of restriction, but claustrophobia still remains a major challenge for radiologic technologists.(1) T——, a registered MRI technologist, told us about his first case after he completed hypnosis training with us.

T—— had positioned the patient on the scanner table and was ready to slide her in, but she was very, very distressed, and her eyes, fixated on the MRI machine, became more and more anxious. She was clearly claustrophobic, and T—— felt sure that this patient would be jumping off the table in the next 10 seconds. He told her, "Listen, I have some relaxation techniques, which I'm very good at. If you can give me 51%, I'll take you the other 49%. Do you want to go for it?" "Oh no. No, no, I can't do it!" she insisted. "That's okay, that's okay," said T——, "but you're pretty upset right now; so how about if you just stay on the table for 5 minutes to calm down. Let me help you relax a little bit, and then if you don't want to have the scan that will be fine. You can just get off the table and go, but at least you won't be starting your day stressed out and you're not coming out of here so upset. If you like the process, you can go into the scanner. If not, I have absolutely no problem with it." He let her know that it was okay to relax and not be concerned about just staying there: "I get paid by the hour, not by the patient," T—— added to relieve any potential reluctance she might have had about inconveniencing the facility by occupying the equipment without getting scanned.

The patient felt T——'s confidence and followed his lead. T—— had the patient breathing deeply in and deeply out, and proceeded with a short induction he had learned in his hypnosis training. The patient calmed down quickly, and was breathing regularly. T—— asked her whether she was feeling relaxed now, and whether she wanted to get off the table and leave now. The patient replied, "No, let's give it a shot," just like T—— knew she would! T—— told her she could take a journey to wherever she wanted to, and he would help her get to her destination. Then T—— went into the adjacent control room. He was no sooner settled there when he heard the patient calling him from inside the scanner. He thought the patient was getting claustrophobic again and walked back into the scanner room. "What's the matter, what's the matter?" he asked. "Oh I'm on that big Carnival Cruise Line now—in a red dress, drinking Chivas Regal. I can feel the wind, T——, I can really feel it. This is wonderful. I don't want it to stop." In her mind, she was totally absorbed in the experience on the cruise ship - all the while she was in the magnet with a power injector hooked up to her, and very confined and in an awkward position. After the procedure she couldn't thank T—— enough for having shown how to get herself through the test. She was pretty proud of herself. ***Case Notes, E. Lang***

What This Case Illustrates Imagining a pleasant experience helps patients forget the immediate stresses of the medical environment and enables cooperation.

Imagery

Imagery replaces a person's attention on the peripheral surroundings and concurrent reality with a focus on past, future, or imagined content. Remembering what you did yesterday, thinking about what you will tomorrow, imagining a pink elephant, describing from memory how your meal tasted, humming a song you heard are all examples of imagery. When you use imagery to help patients through medical encounters, you want their focus on a pleasant scene in which they can become fully absorbed through all of their senses: seeing, hearing, touching, smelling, and tasting.

How to Invite Imagery

One way to structure imagery is to do it interactively—the hypnotized patient tells you where he or she imagines him- or herself to be, and you build on that information. In the earlier years, Dr. Lang's team used to invite patients to "let an image come up," or to imagine where they would rather be or what they would rather be doing. While many patients were able to do this, some expressed reluctance or inability to imagine anything; as if they felt that imagining was not a grownup or macho thing to do. Dr. Lang recalls the case of a young man who was so convinced that he could not imagine anything that the hypnosis practitioner ended up having him describe in great detail the contents of his refrigerator. This definitely was imagery, but way more rudimentary than one would have liked. Some patients, when asked where they would like to go, or what place they like to visit or have always wanted to visit, spontaneously name a place or setting. Some patients however can't decide and go into deliberations and might say, oh, I could go to *X*, or *Y*, or let me think of *Z*. Such critical thinking and rationalizing about where to go interferes with having the conscious mind step in the background and let subconscious choices come up. In such a case you can say: "That is okay. You don't have to decide now. You can enjoy yourself while you just rest here patiently. It will become clearer to you where you might feel comfortable and safe now, or in a moment from now, or in a few moments from now."

Interestingly, the wording in the Study Script 12.1 has never failed to inspire patients to spontaneously initiate imagery for themselves. The script sets the stage with "floating somewhere safe and comfortable, in a bath, a lake, a hot tub, or just floating in space, with each breath deeper and easier." After suggesting that patients, "let a little more tension out of your body as you let your whole body float, safe and comfortable, each breath deeper and easier," patients invariably have answers to the following questions: "Good, now with your eyes closed and remaining in this state of concentration, please describe for me how your body is feeling right now. Where do you imagine yourself being; what is it like? Can you smell the air? Can you see what is around you?" The patients' ability to answer these questions is evidence that they are immersed in their imagery. However, if the patient doesn't answer, you can say, "There is no need to speak out loud or answer me, so just enjoy your experience."

Dr. Laser likes to structure imagery for patients as follows:

After asking the patient an important question, namely, where do you like to go when you want to feel safe and comfortable, Dr. Laser then takes the person to that place.

"You can go there now or in a few minutes from now, and you don't even have to buy a ticket or pack. From your imagination and your imagination alone, you can go there noooooow."

If the patient wants to go to a place he or she hasn't been yet, the last sentence would be replaced by:

"You can create your experience in this beautiful place."

Dr. Laser then uses general information about the named place to build the imagery for the patients while the medical procedure progresses. Dr. Laser uses ideomotor finger signals (See chapter 15, "Ideomotor Signals.") to make sure she remains on track with the patient.

"And yes, being in this comfortable, pleasant, and safe place, you know how to relax here, taking in all the surroundings and magnificent qualities that nature provides, feeling peaceful and safe. And when you are in this safe place, please allow your Yes finger to signal me. Thank you."

Wording is very important. Always ask the patient to suggest the place where he or she likes to go when he or she "wants to feel safe and comfortable." We strongly caution against inviting imagery that brings a patient back to "a happy time" or to childhood. Doing so can lead to your inadvertent age regression of a patient, and you, as the practitioner, have no idea of what happened to the patient during that time. Stage hypnotists sometimes enjoy showing how a person suddenly speaks, writes, and acts like a child. Dr. Lang witnessed this once herself when a stage hypnotist had a group of people behave like youngsters and a young woman suddenly completely disintegrated, cried, and left the stage. Horrifically, the hypnotist would not even help the person with this abreaction—release of tension by recalling trauma. In another incident several years ago, a 40-year old British woman won a court settlement against a stage hypnotist whose routine had reawakened memories of her sexual abuse when she was 8 years old. The reawakening left the woman depressed and suicidal.[(2)] So be careful. Days that may have been exteriorly "happy," could be covering some trauma for the patient, and you do not want to have to treat an abreaction during a procedure. Your goal is to help a patient through a stressful medical encounter. Anchoring a patient in a safe and comfortable place not only aids in preventing an abreaction, but also helps you bring the patient back to this place of comfort and safety should something in the environment trigger an abreaction. This book is designed to help you reach that goal and does not seek to teach or to encourage you to provide psychotherapy.

Where Patients Would Rather Be

Patients tend to pick highly individual imagery that may not necessarily be what the practitioner would choose or find soothing. In a study in 1999, Dr. Lang and colleagues analyzed where patients chose to be in hypnosis during their interventional radiology procedures.[3] Common themes were nature and travel, family and home, and personal skills. Being with loved ones was an important element of imagery for about one quarter of patients. More than half chose passive contemplation, the others were action oriented. While some chose exotic vacations, just as many chose activities or settings that were familiar and over which the patients had control: laying in a recliner, sleeping in bed, canning vegetables while watching TV, working in the woodshop, flying an airplane at night. One person enjoyed floating on clouds with deceased loved ones. In this Midwest sample, few patients spent time at the beach or at rivers. In contrast, on the East Coast, a majority of patients prefer beach scenes. Occasionally patients come up with imagery that may be distasteful to you. It's their choice. If they wish to chase naked maidens in the woods that is okay for them to do; but this is not imagery that you want to aid by structuring interactively. In such cases, just instruct the patients to enjoy their own experience.

Pleasant Imagery

Imagery can be experienced as being within one's body and being absorbed in the situation with all one's senses or from the viewpoint of an observer from a distant perspective. A principle of imagery is that you want to experience good things from within your body and that you want to have bad things outside and away from the body. When patients are in a safe and pleasant environment, you can provide an immediate bodily experience as follows.

"While you are here now (in your living room, Yosemite, on the beach...) in your body, looking out through your eyes, what do you see? Are there any sounds? Can you feel the air on your skin? Is it warm or cool? Are there smells?"

Address all sensory aspects. If you can include in the imagery notions of "down" or "deep" and "deeper," it signals the patient to go down into a deeper trance. Incorporating medical procedure stimuli in the imagery is helpful too. For example if a patient is resting on the beach in the sun and you are ready to cleanse the skin with cold disinfecting solution, you can suggests that there is "a sensation of pleasant coolness—just as when you put on the sunscreen;" or if the gastroenterologist is ready to advance the endoscope through the mouth and throat into the stomach, the patient may be lead to enjoy a sherbet or other favorite meal and swallow bite by bite while tasting all the nuances of the flavors; or may slurp a favorite spaghetti and long slippery noodles gliding down. Sometimes even the most disconcerting sensations can be folded into beautifully imagery, as shown in the following Journal Entry:

JOURNAL ENTRY 18.1

Turbulence in the Air

B—— had completed her research fellowship in the Nonpharmacologic Analgesia Program and was taking a vacation before starting work in another hospital. She sent me an excited e-mail about her flight from Jamaica to Philadelphia. Next to her fiancé sat a girl, who started to panic because of some turbulence. She was crying and shaking, and her parents were not able to calm her down. Finally B—— changed seats with her fiancé, introduced herself and started hypnotizing the girl. Since they were in bad weather and the plane started to shake significantly, B—— suggested that that the girl go back to Jamaica to the beach and go snorkeling. As the girl could feel the motion of the waves (actually the motion of the airplane, which was shaking) and as she could see thousands of fish, one of them was diving deeper and deeper and deeper. The girl became so deeply hypnotized that she was sitting relaxed and with her eyes closed in her seat for about an hour. The landing was pretty rough, too, but now the girl was on her boat sailing slowly back to the beach, which she reached as soon as the plane landed. Her parents were totally impressed. They told B—— that they have never seen their daughter that calm and relaxed in a plane and that they wished B—— could go on every vacation with them. B——'s fiancé, who had followed her work in hypnosis, but had been a bit of a skeptic said: "I believed you that it would work, but I didn't expect this." ***Journal Notes, E. Lang***

Distressing Imagery

Sometimes patients may describe spontaneously how they feel in terms of distressing imagery: "As if vultures are coming down to get me," "Like a little field mouse surrounded by big cats," "As if a gray mule is kicking my back," "Like a piece of red meat with a butcher knife all the way through." When patients offer distressing imagery, your goal is to dissociate the patient from the threatening experience. It such cases you want patients to see themselves from a distance (like on a screen) and either remove the offending elements or convert those elements into supportive and protective pleasant imagery. For example, if the vultures are coming down to get the patient, you can have the vultures fly off into the distance, turn them into beautiful geese who drop their softest down feathers and a beautiful down blanket comes to wrap the patient in a soft bed of comfort, tranquility, and protection. The patient then can experience being wrapped into this wonderful down blanket that keeps out all that is not helpful, and into which the patient can sink deeper and deeper. The little field mouse can grow big and strong into Mighty Mouse and chase the cats away. Mighty Mouse then can enjoy the barnyard in her favorite spot where it is warm and cozy and just right and very safe.

Key Points to Remember

- Imagining a pleasant experience helps patients forget the immediate stresses of the medical environment and enables cooperation.
- Imagery replaces a person's attention on peripheral surroundings and concurrent reality with a focus on past, future, or imagined content.
- Always ask the patient to suggest the place where he or she likes to go "where you feel safe and comfortable," and avoid inviting imagery that brings a patient back to "a happy time" or to childhood, which could trigger an abreaction.
- Using words such as "down," "deep,'" and "deeper," helps deepen trance.
- Pleasant imagery should be an in-body experience during which the patient can take in the imagery with all senses.
- Distressing imagery should be viewed from the distance and the offending elements removed or converted into protective and supportive pleasant images.
- Your goal is to help a patient through a stressful medical encounter. This book is designed to help you reach that goal and does not seek to teach or to encourage you to provide psychotherapy.

Opportunities to Practice

At your next break close your eyes and imagine a place where you would rather be and focus the sights, sounds, feelings, smells, and tastes of the place. Make sure you include at least one element in your imagery from each sensory category and fully associate yourself with the experience. You can do this without a formal induction for self-hypnosis, but at the end, do a formal reorientation by counting backwards from, 3... rolling up your closed eyes, 2...taking a breath in, and 1...feeling, refreshed, awake, and eyes wide open.

CHAPTER 19

Managing Anxiety and Distress

Case 19.1 The Stand-up Comedian

A well made-up, serious, but also scared looking woman was awaiting a tube placement procedure. The patient's intestines were badly scarred as a result of the many abdominal surgeries she had experienced, and she was to receive a feeding tube that would circumvent the blockage in her gut. She agreed to have the procedure done with hypnosis, but was very anxious and explained how nervous she was. Dr. Lang knew that it would be very difficult to proceed with an induction until she could first address what caused the patient's distress. After quick consideration, Dr. Lang chose to use the Parts-Model approach, which is based on the theory that we all have different parts or aspects to our personalities and that when one part senses danger it can produce behavior that may appear externally unhelpful to the person but is grounded in the best intention for the individual. Dr. Lang asked the patient: "Can you tell me where in your body this feeling is coming from?" The patient pointed to her upper chest/neck junction and said, "Right here. It is as if it is choking me." Dr. Lang suggested, "Okay, you know this part that is causing the sensation is a part of you; and as such it has a good intention. So why don't you move it outside of you and ask it what is its good intention? You may even ask the part if it has a name." The patient replied that she could do this and also named the part. The part was telling her that it wanted her to go through the procedure safely and to get well again. Dr. Lang suggested that the patient thank the part for its good intentions, and to also thank the part for all the hard work it had done throughout the patient's life. The part had gotten her though a lot of hardship and challenges and that it really deserved great thanks. The patient thanked the part.

Dr. Lang next suggested that the patient also ask the part if it would be okay to take on a new job description; in fact to get a promotion; and to see if it could help the patient to achieve the goal of going safely through the procedure, but without giving her the feeling she had been experiencing. The patient indicated that the part agreed with that, and that it also wanted her to bring joy and laughter to people. The patient then told the medical team that for a short time in her past, she had wanted to become a stand-up comedian and actually had performed in some clubs. Now, she told the team, she would like to guide them through the procedure by giving them some laughs and a good time. That settled, the patient was brought to the procedure room, at ease with herself as she entertained everyone. She made us laugh while being prepped and then quietly and smiling, let us go on. The procedure continued without problems. ***Case Notes, E. Lang***

What This Case Illustrates Anything that is causing the patient distress should be brought outside of and away from the patient. Making an ally of what is bothering the patient is particularly helpful. The Parts-Model is one of several ways to achieve this goal.

Strategies for Distress Management

Anxiety prior to a procedure is a predictor of intraoperative pain, anxiety, need for medications, and length of procedure.(1) The first step in minifying anxiety is simply to ask patients to take a deep breath in...and as they do, to take in relaxation...and with their breath out...to breathe out any tension or anything else that is not helpful. A few repeats of this directed breathing may be all you need to do.

Some patients spontaneously come up with an image for how they feel. For example, the patient may say, "I feel like I'm caught in a cold dungeon with no way out." When a patient offers such imagery, you neutralize and transform it as described in chapter 18, "Imagery." Distressing imagery can be neutralized and/or moved away through several approaches. For example, you can ask the patient to describe the color, shape, etc. of the distressing image. Then have them alter these images characteristics and send the image far away. Distressing imagery can be moved away and/or neutralized in size (for example, made smaller), color (for example, burning red may be turned into calming gray or white), temperature (generally, pleasantly warm or cooling instead of burning or freezing), and ability to affect the patient adversely. How you can convert the patient's distressing imagery is shown in the following Journal Entry:

JOURNAL ENTRY 19.1

A Ball of Fire

The patient was deathly afraid of needles and dreaded the hurt of the inevitable upcoming shot, but she was barely able to tolerate the pain in her lower back. She had nowhere else to turn, but to this procedure. We secured her position on the table, having her sit up, so that the doctor could aim at the correct level of the spine, and I guided her into trance. The patient spontaneously described her pain. She said it was as if there was a red ball of fire hitting her back. I suggested she could move the ball up, up, and away to a mountaintop, very high up and very far away. She did and acknowledged that she accomplished it. I then asked her to change the color of the ball from red to a more soothing color; and to move it farther away again and again until it was a tiny dot, almost invisible. The patient made these changes to the ball, and she continued to cooperatively assist the doctor in the medical procedure. The doctor injected several locations and the woman sat quietly and comfortably through it all. I also told the patient, that from her memory and her memory alone, she could recall this feeling of ease and control over her pain on her own, and doing so would become a skill that could help her whenever she needed it. ***Journal Notes, E. Laser***

The Parts Model

The Part-of-Self tool can be used to address over-reactivity or "acting-out" of an affect[2] and is based on Ego State Therapy.[3] The idea is that individuals are all comprised of different parts or ego-states from varying developmental levels and roles in life. A person's parts may include a child, a teenager, a professional adult, a spouse, a neighbor, a member of a social group, etc., and normally all are integrated in the overall personality. The premise continues that each of these parts have their functions in protecting the individual. However, sometimes the only way a part that senses a threat can express its protective purpose is by producing behaviors that externally look anything but helpful.

For our purposes here in *Patient Sedation Without Medication,* we will not fully explore Ego State Therapy, but we do want to offer just a small piece from it to use in a safe way to help patients through procedures. We use it mainly when patients are too distraught by their upset feelings to even begin an induction. When asking patients to address the part that is causing the problem, you can use the Parts Model as illustrated in case 19.1 or the following or similar language:

> Go to the part that is creating the feeling of being scared (or that is giving you this feeling). Take a body scan and you will feel the part signal you—you might feel a flutter or a

squeeze or heaviness or something similar, and when you feel the feeling in your body; let us know where it is. *(Either a nod of the head or an ideomotor signal will indicate it.)* Okay, thank you. Ask the part to come forward so that you can see it in front of you. You can hold it in your hands or look at it. Now give the part a voice. And now, ask the part what it is that it wants for you? It has good intentions and it will tell you. Ask the part if it would enjoy helping you do another job? Tell the part you appreciate its positive intention and loyalty over the years. It never even asked for a raise. Now we need the part's help to protect you in this new experience during your procedure. Can we count on the part to help? Thank the part again. Just let yourself relax now. The part will help you stay well.

The Pile of Sand

For some patients gradual stress relief works quite well. When performing breast biopsies, during which patients are particularly anxious, Dr. Lang favors the gradual stress relief techniques such as an adapted Pile of Sand Induction.(4) This technique came in particularly handy on the East coast where patients love to go to the beach. Luckily, patients don't have to love the beach to benefit from this induction; you can always adjust the location so that patients who are afraid of water don't get too close to it. You begin by asking the patient to build a pile of things bothering him or her; to just take all his or her worries and all those feelings that are unhelpful and to just pile them up, build them into a huge pile, like a pile of sand. Encourage the patient to have the pile grow bigger and bigger by just throwing on everything that comes to mind. Tell the patient to pile it on with abandon, the more the better, to really build the pile up. Tell the patient to make it as high as it needs to be (one patient told Dr. Lang, it had reached heaven). When the patient feels he or she has piled everything possible on, have him or her tell you. The patient can nod, or give an ideomotor signal (See chapter 15, "Ideomotor Signals). Next, have the patient think of the waves of the ocean (or whichever body of water is appropriate for the patient) coming gently up onto the shore against the pile and then rolling gently back into the ocean. Tell the patient that each wave in brings relaxation, and each wave out carries a bit more of the "sand" pile away with it, and regardless of how high the pile is, the power of the gentle waves is such that the pile will become smaller and smaller. Each wave brings in more relaxation and each wave carries out and washes away more and more of the pile—wave by wave—until the entire pile of worries and unhelpful feelings is gone.

Another technique for the gradual relief of stress in patients is the Red Balloon Induction. Following is the script for this technique.

Script 19.1 The Red Balloon

Imagine a meadow, filled with gorgeous colorful flowers, blue, yellow, red, and lavender, all of its vibrancy shone far into the distance. You are lured to this gorgeous, glorious place, and as you walk closer and closer, you see a huge red balloon. As you continue to come closer, you realize that the red balloon is tied to a huge basket and has another basket within. And now, you see that the outer basket is weighted down by sandbags. You remove the inner basket and hear within yourself, that you are to place all your worries, self doubts, fears, complaints, disenchantments, and all other negative beliefs into the inner basket. You have all the time you need. As you face the basket, you soon place every feeling that you want to unload, into the container. As you do, you begin to feel less constraint and burdened. Now, imagine putting the filled inner basket back into the outer basket, and then imagine your hands untying the ropes that hold the outer basket to the weights, and as each rope is untied, a sandbag falls to the ground. As the sandbags fall, you now have the power to let go, to release, and unburden your inner self. You have now gained enjoyment in life, and begin a new day. As the red balloon lifts the container away, you can actually feel the burdens of self-doubt, anxieties, fears, worries, and all negative beliefs, lifted from your shoulders. As the balloon continues to raise high in the sky, finally into the universe, you can only see a faint dot, a tiny hue of red that fades away in the sunset. From now on, you can recreate this image from your memory, and continue to enjoy life with a new positive approach feeling relieved and refreshed. ***End of Script 19.1***

The Split Screen Technique

The Study Script (See chapter 12, "Hypnosis by Script,") describes a method for distress management, called the *Split Screen Technique.* One advantage of this technique over the use of an imagery process is that you do not need to come up with any of the solutions for the patient. The idea of the Split Screen Technique is that you first have the patient picture in his or her mind a screen like a movie screen or TV screen, or just imagine a piece of blue sky; you can even have the patient imagine a pleasant scene on it. Then you have the patient picture a large piece of blue screen divided in half. Have the patient picture what is bothering him or her on the left side of the screen. This action projects the source of the patient's distress away—still able to be viewed, but no longer experienced. As the patient describes the scene on the left you can say "Hmm" a few times and listen attentively. Next, you suggest that the patient work on the solution to what is bothering him or her by projecting the solution on the right side of the screen. If the patient cannot come up with a solution for the right side of the screen—ask what he or she would recommend someone else in the same situation do—no one has ever failed this one.

The Split Screen Technique can be examined in light of sensory preferences signals associated with eye position as discussed in chapter 6, "Interpreting Eye Position." In chapter 6, you learned that in principle, people tend to move their eyes to the left when accessing memory and to the right when constructing content. So the brain is primed to the idea that what is shown on the left is "old and done" and what is seen on the right is "new and future."

Key Points to Remember

- It is important to address patient's distress and anxiety early on—otherwise they will have a difficult time entering trance.
- Anything that is causing the patient distress should be brought outside of and away from the patient.
- Asking patients to take a deep breath in, and as they do to take in relaxation, and with their breath out to blow out any tension or anything else that is not helpful, may be all you need to do to relax the patient.
- When anxiety assumes imagery, the goal is to move the distressing imagery away. Change its color, temperature, or size, have it carried away, and if possible convert it into something more beneficial.
- The parts model can be used when patients are so anxious that they can't relax enough to enter trance.
- The Pile of Sand and The Red Balloon are examples of techniques that gradually relieve distress.
- The Split Screen Technique is helpful and straightforward in addressing anxiety, worries, and distress since the patient comes up with all the solutions.

Opportunities to Practice

Next time you get stressed, see which of the techniques presented in this chapter work for you: breathing the tension out, associating an image and changing it, using the parts model, Pile of Sand, Red Balloon, or Split Screen.

CHAPTER 20

Managing Pain

Case 20.1 The Strained Ankle

Dr. Lang was on her way to meet a former colleague for lunch in the hospital. She had strained her ankle two days earlier and limped to the appointment well aware of the remaining pain. The lunch was pure pleasure—a great opportunity to reminisce and consider some future collaboration. The colleague then took Dr. Lang on a walk through the newly renovated hospital wing and offices in an adjacent building—quite a tour. Throughout their journey, they ran into many common acquaintances and it was wonderful greeting everyone; often stopping to talk a little and quickly exchange catch-up information. Starting to walk back home, Dr. Lang realized how easy the walking had been going during the tour and that she had all but forgotten about her ankle. And with that thought—the pain was back! ***Case Notes, E. Lang***

What This Case Illustrates Focusing the mind on something other than one's pain can greatly reduce the hurt or even remove it from awareness.

Effect of Hypnosis on Pain

The experience of pain is subjective. Hypnosis helps with pain management in two ways: by taking the mind off what is hurting and by changing how the stimulus is processed in the brain. The experience of pain has three components:

- **Sensory component:** How intense a stimulus is registered
- **Cognitive component:** What the stimulus is interpreted to be
- **Affective component:** What this means psychologically

The affective component involves emotional reactions. As you may have experienced, physical stimuli of identical intensity can be experienced as more or less hurtful depending on the situation. For example, the physical insults one may experience during a backpacking trip or while learning how to snowboard are most likely to be interpreted as part of the recreational fun and quite acceptable. The same stimuli, in a less enjoyable context, might be interpreted as torturous and unacceptable. As Dr. David Spiegel likes to put it, "The strain in the pain is in the brain." Hypnosis can take the hurt out of the pain by altering the overall processing of potentially painful stimuli, in particular by moderating their affective component.[1-3] Another mechanism by which hypnosis decreases the perception of pain is by the reduction of anxiety—a potent predictor of intraprocedural distress and pain.[4]

Through our clinical trials, we became aware of an interesting phenomenon: under standard care conditions, patients' pain increases steadily over time—regardless of the amount of medication they receive and regardless of the type of procedure they undergo.[5-7] When in doubt, the unconscious mind interprets a situation as negative.[8] In light of this tendency, it follows that the ambiguity of the stimuli a patient experiences when first placed on a procedure table tends to cause the patient to interpret the stimuli as painful—even when they are not. Furthermore, once one has experienced one stimulus as painful, one tends to experience subsequent ones as also painful—even when they are not.[9] We discovered in the trials that we could interrupt this usual mechanism of steady increase of pain right from the beginning simply by reading the patient a hypnotic script.

According to the criteria of the American Psychological Association Clinical Psychology Division, there is sufficient scientific evidence to consider hypnosis an efficacious and specific treatment for pain, which shows superiority to pills and placebo.[10] This is good news for nearly everyone. It is true that ability to experience hypnosis varies with the individual. Only about 10-20% patients can go into such a deep trance that one could perform open surgery on them without any anesthesia.[11; 12] Fortunately, for less invasive procedures, the majority of patients have enough hypnotic ability to be helped by hypnotic adjuncts.[13] These facts make a patient's potential hypnotizability a moot point for the use of *Patient Sedation Without Medication.* We, therefore, do not measure hypnotizability because doing so would unnecessarily take extra time and also could set up counterproductive standards and expectations.

Approaches of Hypnotic Pain Management

Patients may experience hypnotic analgesia just by using relaxation techniques and self-hypnosis. Often, as in the example of case 20.1 "The Strained Ankle," just diverting the patient's attention from what is hurting can be enough to bring relief. You can give patients specific suggestions to help the diversion along. When about to administer potentially painful stimuli, you might have the patient focus on a competing sensation. For example, when you give the local anesthetic, you can say to the patient, "Just focus on a sensation of coolness or a delicious sensation of tingling, and numbness that is spreading to all the areas it needs to." If a patient is already in pain from a preexisting condition when being placed on the procedure table, you can suggest that he or she imagine putting a hot pack or ice on the painful spot.

Dr. Marcia Greenleaf, an experienced psychologist and hypnotherapist, describes how her father, Dr. Selig Finkelstein—a dentist—once told a child, whose front teeth along with parts of the adjacent nerves had been knocked out, to imagine his left hand was deep into a bucket of ice cubes.(14) Dr. Finkelstein then suggested that the child raise his left hand when it felt numb from the cold of the ice and then to transfer the numbness of his left hand to his right hand. Dr. Finkelstein further instructed the child that once his right hand was also numb, he should transfer the numbness to his mouth. This episode is an example of a form of *glove anesthesia,* in which the patient learns to develop insensitivity to pain in one body part and then applies this insensitivity to another distant body part.

Another approach is to have patients focus very attentively on a different body part, distant from the pain site. Attention can also be diverted away from a painful procedure stimulus towards a manageable task. For example, ask the patient to tightly squeeze the thumb against the ring finger of the right hand while you place an IV in the left arm. During a prolonged bolus injection of contrast medium for lower extremity arteriography, the patient can be instructed to "breathe in... breathe out...breathe in...breathe out...," in a rhythmic fashion while the images of the lower extremity are obtained.

Still another option is to use the breathing technique described in the "Progressive Muscle Relaxation Scripts 17.1 and 17.2," In these scripts, patients are instructed to imagine that they are inhaling relaxation and comfort with each breath in, and told to allow that breath to focus on the very spot of their body that they would like to feel even more relaxed. Patients are further encouraged to allow their exhaled breath to go right to that spot, and to breath any tension right out through the skin at that spot.

You can help divert some potential patient perceptions of pain throughout the procedure by staying focused on the language you use to announce procedure stimuli. Replacing "pain" with "sensation" or "feeling" diverts from a focus on hurt. As discussed in chapter 8, "Avoiding Negative Suggestions," it is important to use imagery with neutral or positive connotations to announce procedure stimuli. For example, rather than warning that the bolus of contrast medium you are going to inject will feel "as if a bomb is exploding inside you," (poor choice of words) you can instead predict, "a soothing feeling of warmth that will spread throughout your body" (much better choice of words).

An important reminder: As indicated in chapter 21, "Stabilizing Physiology," one really has to indicate the exact target, not just a direction when asking the patient to make physiological self-adjustments. In other words, be specific. Don't tell patients "you will feel warmer and warmer (or cooler and cooler)," because they will do just that. Instead, be specific and suggest limits. You might say, "You may feel warmth. You will be able to regulate how warm it will be...just think of something cooling and dilute the warmth to a degree that feels just right for you." You can suggest cool spring water, snow, frozen yogurt with hot chocolate, tea on ice, or anything that suits the patient's imagination and current imagery.

The following journal entry is another example of integrating upcoming procedure stimuli into the patient's experience.

JOURNAL ENTRY 20.1

Ed Goes to Alaska

Ed had a blood clot in his leg and was to receive an inferior vena cava filter, a small metal umbrella that is placed in the large vein draining the lower part of the body so that the clot will not travel into the patient's lungs should it become loose. For the procedure, an access in the groin vein is opened with increasingly larger dilators until the introducer capsule for the filter—a device, about the size of a small finger, can be inserted. I was going to assist the patient with hypnosis during the procedure and decided to use imagery.

I asked Ed where he would like to go, if he could go anywhere. Spontaneously, he answered, "Alaska." So, once he was settled on the procedure table, we headed north. Ed didn't have to pack or buy a ticket; he only had to go into trance. He did, and so his Alaska visit began. Ed didn't have a care in the world. He was visiting Alaska and was able to tell me what his senses were experiencing. Ed saw lodges and igloos and was eager to go into one; so he did. Inside the lodge, Ed met many people and was invited to be part of an ongoing celebration Meanwhile, as the surgical procedure progressed, I realized that Ed may be feeling pulling and tugging or a sort of bumping sensation as Dr. Lang and her assistant pushed the device into place. I incorporated these sensations into Ed's imagery telling him that it was pretty crowded with everyone having come from near and far for this event, and sometimes people might bump into one another; its very close and they enjoy bumping up against each other, because its all in the game. It's a natural part of being together and being comfortable. Ed was smiling. In fact, when he woke up, he was still smiling. He really enjoyed Alaska. The procedure went well. ***Journal Notes, E. Laser***

Changing the meaning of the procedure stimulus for the patient can have profound impact on his or her experience of pain. This holds particularly true for patients in whom treatment is associated with destruction of tumor tissue such as during chemoembolization of tumors. During this process, doctors inject anti-cancer drugs directly into the blood vessels that are feeding the tumor. They additionally place other materials—embolic agents—in the blood vessels to mechanically block the blood supply to the tumor. These measures, in effect, kill the tumor tissue. Patients who associate the ensuing pain with dying tumor tissue better accept the sensation. Keeping the patient informed about the progress of the procedure in terms of the desired outcome enhances acceptability of intermittent potentially painful stimuli.

One more technique to consider is the imaginary control device. Some patients may benefit from an imagery scenario in which they control a switch or button or dial that controls the pain. For example, a patient can choose to turn his or her own endorphin "pharmacy" on and off when needed, to provide comfort and ease pain.

Concurrent Use of Sedatives and Narcotics

In the beginning of our studies, we had some concerns that the concurrent use of pharmaceuticals could alter the ability of patients to follow hypnotic suggestions. This, fortunately, has been disproved in the ensuring clinical trials. Patients like to have a pharmaceutical "safety-blanket" if they are to engage in moderate or more invasive procedures. In other words, they want to be assured that they can have drugs, if and when they want them. For appropriate invasive procedures, we therefore give patients a button to push when they want to receive medication, and within limits of safety, they do receive it. The button obviates the need for patients to explain why they "need" the meds and enhances trust. This method also obviates the possibility that patients would hold back from requesting medication so as not to disappoint the person who is helping them with hypnosis. Offering the patient the possibility of both medication and hypnosis gives the patient choices right upfront. With those choices comes a sense of control that in itself has a beneficial aspect for the patient.

Although we do also offer patients the choice of pharmaceuticals, it has been our experience—as well as the experience of other investigators—that the use of hypnosis greatly reduces the amount of medications needed, and thus, also reduces the number of associated drug-induced complications.

No Room for Guilt

It is important to remember that all you can offer patients is the help they need to help themselves. You cannot force and you cannot guarantee. You can guide patients, but they will have to want to cooperate. And also with a patient's best effort, pain may not always go down to zero. Thus if a patient is not completely pain-free or doesn't seem to respond to hypnosis, you should not feel guilty. On the other hand, when things go especially well and the patient experiences a very deep trance, you cannot take all the credit either.

Keep your goals objective and reasonable. A reduction of pain to an acceptable level is in itself a great achievement. You can be assured that your patient would be ultimately worse off if you had not offered *Patient Sedation Without Medication* techniques.

JOURNAL ENTRY 20.2

Putting the Outcome in Perspective

We conducted our first prospective randomized study of Nonpharmacologic Analgesia (that is how we referred to the techniques of *Patient Sedation Without Medication* at the time) and had come close to the final 240th patient of the study. We just had experienced a run of "difficult" patients, and I started to wonder what the final data analysis would show. Then a young patient participated and was randomized to receive hypnosis during her procedure. Prior to this admission, she had had multiple hospital stays, many surgeries, therapeutic ups-and-downs, and was greatly sensitized to the stresses of the medical environment. What's more, her pain threshold was a very low. All of these factors contributed to delays in the process, including that the hypnosis induction took longer than the technologist team would have liked.

The case completed well, but afterwards one of the technologists began complaining, loudly, that hypnosis was a waste of time. To answer the question of why she thought that, the technologist offered as evidence that this last patient did not become fully relaxed and certainly wasn't entirely pain free. After allowing the technologist to vent, I asked her to recall a time when she had this very patient for an earlier procedure outside of the study and asked her to remember how that procedure went for the patient—and for her. Only then did the technologist remember that at that earlier procedure, the patient had been crying and trying to get up from the table for half an hour with this technologist holding the patient half upright in her arms and trying to calm her during the entire procedure. This earlier traumatic response by the patient had happened despite considerable amounts of medications the patient had received for that procedure. From the perspective of this earlier experience, the patient's present experience with hypnosis although admittedly not "fully relaxed," or "entirely pain free," was a huge success. ***Journal Notes, E. Lang***

Although the above "Journal Entry," is an individual case, data analysis showed that this case was representative of the broad picture of these incidents.(7) The patients in the hypnosis group had significantly less pain, less anxiety, less need for drugs, fewer complications; and, in addition, were done 17 minutes faster than those in the control group. Thus, proving the additional point that hypnosis helps without adding excessive time to the procedure schedule. The data from these trials gave us the knowledge and proof that we needed. From then on we have been confident that patients do benefit greatly from procedure hypnosis and that regardless of how it may seem at the time—patients are ultimately better off with the hypnosis option than without it.

Key Points to Remember

- Focusing the mind on something other than one's pain can greatly reduce the hurt or even remove it from awareness.
- Pain perception has sensory, cognitive, and affective aspects.

- Hypnosis helps with pain management not only by taking the mind off from what is hurting but also by changing how pain is processed in the brain.
- When in doubt, the unconscious mind interprets a situation as negative.
- For hypnotic pain management you can use suggestions that focus on a different sensation, on a different body part, on a manageable task, on a breathing technique that has the patient breathe the pain right through the skin, or suggest glove anesthesia or similar transferable mode of numbness to the painful area.
- You can integrate procedure stimuli into the patient's imagery.
- Concurrent use of sedatives doesn't interfere with the patients' ability to engage in procedure hypnosis.
- While only a fraction of patients are sufficiently hypnotizable to undergo open surgery without anesthetics, practically all patients can benefit from Sedation Without Medication.
- You have not failed if your patient experiences pain. You can be assured that without your assistance, they would have done much worse. There is no room for guilt.

Opportunities to Practice

- Choose one of the following approaches for managing pain: have the patient focus on a competing sensation, imagine applying heat or cold to the pain, focus on a different body part, focus on a manageable task, use breathing techniques, and use an imaginary pain control button. Plan how you will present this approach to patients and use it at the next patient opportunity. When you are comfortable with that approach, choose another.
- Think of imagery you can use in your area to describe potentially painful stimuli.

CHAPTER 21
Stabilizing Physiology

Case 21.1 Raise the Blood Pressure

As part of a biliary procedure Dr. Lang was performing, she placed catheters through the patient's skin and liver across a narrow spot in the patient's bile ducts. Dr. Lang noted that the patient's baseline blood pressure was around 100/60 mm Hg. The patient had received some IV drugs for relaxation and pain management, and Dr. Laser had assisted with hypnosis. The patient's blood pressure decreased to about 90/60 mm Hg. Dr. Lang would have preferred to have the blood pressure a little higher to have some reserve for potential procedure-related drops. However, she hesitated to use the standard measures for increasing blood pressure, such as infusing more fluids through the IV or giving medications because the patient looked quite comfortable. Instead, Dr. Lang asked Dr. Laser to get the patient's pressure up. Dr. Laser approached the patient and gave her the hypnotic suggestion to, "raise your blood pressure." The case went on, and when watching the monitors, Dr. Lang noticed that the systolic blood pressure had reached 145 mm Hg and was still rising. Dr. Lang told Dr. Laser to get the systolic pressure to 120 mm Hg and hold it there. Dr. Laser suggested to the patient that she go into her brain and look at the dial which regulates her systolic blood pressure and set it at 120 mm Hg. The patient complied, and her blood pressure stabilized exactly at 120 mm Hg, to the dot. ***Case Notes, E. Laser***

What This Case Illustrates When suggesting changes in patient physiology, such as in blood pressure, to patients in trance, it is important to be very specific. The subconscious mind takes things very literally, and amazing as it may seem, accurately generates the precise suggested outcome.

Suggestions Need To Be Specific

Case 21.1, "Raise the Blood Pressure," illustrates the importance of being specific and precise when suggesting to patients in hypnosis that they affect their physiology. This case was the first time Dr. Lang had incorporated such suggestions into a procedure and quickly learned that saying, "raise the blood pressure," was not specific enough. One really has to indicate the exact target, not just a direction. Dr. Lang has since successfully used specific suggestions for blood pressure to get the precise increase or decrease that is needed. Other physiological self-adjustments can also be made using hypnotic suggestions, but during procedures and in surgery one should never rely solely on hypnosis to restore patients' stability. A medical team must always be prepared for all eventualities and always have the appropriate drugs and resuscitation equipment at the ready and know how to use them.

Stabilizing Physiology with Hypnosis

We have good news to share. The very act of using self-hypnotic relaxation techniques stabilizes blood pressure and heart rate for patients during medical procedures. This stabilization happens even when the practitioner makes no hypnotic suggestions specifically to bring about this effect. Dr. Lang and colleagues demonstrated this phenomena in three large prospective randomized studies: The Lancet study in 2000 evaluated 241 patients undergoing catheterizations of their blood vessels for procedures on their kidneys: Larger fluctuations in blood pressure and/or heart rate occurred in only 1 of 82 hypnosis patients compared to 12 of 79 standard care patients, and in 10 of 80 patients in the attention control group.[1] Intrigued by these findings, Dr. Lang's group wondered whether the data would also hold up for procedures that are more invasive and associated with hemodynamic disturbances. To explore the possibility, the group assessed patients having tumor embolizations where the blood supply to tumors is blocked off to devitalize the tumor. The tumor tissue begins to die while the patients are still in the procedure suite. Dr. Lang's group halted this study when it became evident that there were significantly greater—and very high—rates of adverse events, including concerning drops or rises in blood pressure and heart beat irregularities in the empathy control group (31 of 65 patients, 48%) as compared to the hypnosis group (8 of 66 patients, 12%)![2]

One could explain reduced adverse event rates during procedures performed with hypnosis by a reduced need for medications that counteract anxiety and pain, but that also depress blood pressure, heart rate, and breathing. Reduced need for drugs, however, can only partially explain the reduced adverse event rate because the beneficial effect of hypnosis is still present when this factor is taken out of the equation.[1]

Hypnosis also results in a more favorable heart rate variability profile.[3-6] Heart rate variability measures the beat-to-beat changes in heart rate going along with the rhythm of a person's autonomous nervous system. Its profile is considered a predictor of cardiovascular risk.[7; 8] We hypothesize that the more favorable profile under hypnosis allows the patient to respond to environmental or internal changes quicker with a series of fine adjustments. These continuous fine adjustments eliminate the need for big, sudden swings in blood pressure or heart rate as the body attempts to restore equilibrium. It is, to a large extent, for this stabilizing effect that Dr. Lang prefers to perform her interventional radiology cases using hypnosis. Many other professionals have begun to share this preference. A nurse, who specializes in breast biopsies, confided that she "loves sedation without medication because ever since her training, none of her patients faint anymore."

Immunization Against Cold

Body temperature is another factor that can be affected by hypnosis. Procedure rooms tend to be kept cool for optimal function of the computer equipment. Since surgeons and team members often are dressed in poorly breathable gowns and sometimes lead aprons, they tend to be warmer than the patient who is naked under a sheet. Also anxiety tends to give people "cold feet" figuratively and literally.

It is difficult to enter hypnosis when one is shivering or uncomfortably cold in a room. In these cases, one can have the patient imagine a warm bath, Jacuzzi, or being warmed by the sunshine or warm blanket and warmed just to the right temperature. Dr. Laser's technique, after induction, is to ask the patient to go to the part of him- or herself that regulates his or her body temperature, and to ask the ideomotor signals (See chapter 15, "Ideomotor Signals") to indicate when that part responds. Then, Dr. Laser asks the patient to adjust the internal temperature gage to a comfortable setting, throughout the procedure. Dr. Laser asks that the patient to allow his or her Yes finger to signal her when the patient has accomplished the task.

When using this technique, remember to watch for the ideomotor signal that will indicate that the patient has adjusted his or her temperature to a comfortable setting; and when you see the signal, anchor the patient in that state by giving him or her a gentle but firm touch on the shoulder (See chapter 7, "Touching in the Medical Environment").

Preparation for Heat from Radiographic Contrast Medium Boluses

Contrast medium used for injection during vascular study can elicit feelings of intense warmth. To immunize the patient against this rush of warmth, for example while studying the lower extremities, you can announce the injection by saying, "You might feel a sensation of agreeable warmth spreading all the way down into your toes...and you can regulate the temperature to the level of warmth that feels best to you. You can mix in as much cool as you like to have a perfect mixture." Another option to use instead, or in addition to this invitation to regulate the effect of the injection, is to integrate temperature adjustments into the patient's imagery as illustrated in the following Journal Entry.

JOURNAL ENTRY 21.1

Too Close to the Sun

A patient with poor blood supply to her legs was having an angiogram. We had used the Study Script induction (See chapter 12, "Hypnosis by Script") and she was floating on clouds in the sky. After the contrast medium injection, she said, "Wow, I guess I must have floated too close to the sun. It got really hot." We suggested that with the next injection she should direct the cloud to float just the right distance from the sun so that she could enjoy the warmth, and be neither too cold nor too hot, but just right. Fortunately, the patient was able to do just that with the following injections and remained comfortable throughout the procedure. ***Journal Notes, E. Lang***

Key Points to Remember

- It is important to be specific and precise when suggesting to patients in hypnosis that they affect their physiology because the subconscious mind takes your suggestions literally.

- Patients in hypnosis are hemodynamically more stable during medical procedures even when you don't give specific suggestions to that extent.
- During procedures and in surgery one should not rely solely on hypnosis to restore patient stability. A medical team must always be prepared for all eventualities and always have the appropriate drugs and resuscitation equipment at the ready and know how to use them.
- Patients who are cold have a hard time entering hypnosis or being able to relax. You can help them get to and anchor them to a place that has just the right temperature.
- You can use imagery that entails dials or regulators in the brain that produce the exact target; you can also integrate temperature adjustments into the patient's imagery.

Opportunities to Practice

- When you have a hard time falling asleep and notice you have cold feet, present yourself imagery that brings just the right amount of blood flow to your feet.
- When you encounter a patient who is cold, provide him or her with a warmed blanket and suggest that the patient warm up to a comfortable level; and if you don't have a blanket use appropriate imagery and anchoring.

CHAPTER 22

Reorientation

Case 22.1 Not Just a Nap

During a hypnosis workshop Dr. Lang attended, a psychologist presented a case from his psychotherapy practice. He showed a video of part of a hypnotic intervention with the patient. At the end of the approximately 40 minutes of hypnosis, the psychologist reoriented the patient by counting backward from ten to one, having the patient become more and more alert as the counting came closer and closer to zero. On the count of three, he had the patient start to move; with the count of two, he had the patient stretch; and on the count of one, he told the patient to have his eyes open, be fully alert, and be delighted with his experience.

The patient opened his eyes on the last suggestion and looked around slowly becoming fully alert. The psychologist asked the patient for feedback about the hypnotic experience. The patient response was, "I really can't say." The patient insisted that he had apparently just fallen asleep during the attempted induction and had a short nap during the session. The patient said he was sorry that the hypnosis didn't work for him. When asked why he thought he had awoken right at the moment that the psychologist had suggested he open his eyes, the patient was at a loss to explain it other than "coincidence". He was also puzzled to learn that a full 40 minutes had passed. To the patient, it had seemed like a really short nap. ***Case Notes, E. Lang***

What This Case Illustrates Patients can develop amnesia for having experienced hypnosis. Hypnosis also induces time distortion.

Posthypnotic Amnesia

Some patients may not remember that they experienced a hypnotic trance, when indeed they did, and explain what happened as a dream or sleep. This is what happened to the patient in the case 22.1, above. This amnesia can also extend to what happened during trance. Interestingly, patients who report pain during hypnosis tend to forget about the pain afterwards or remember the pain as less severe than they reported it to be during the stimulation.[(2)] This phenomenon is helpful when patients have to undergo repeat procedures. Their vague memory causes them to expect less distress during the next procedure, and that expectation becomes a self-fulfilling prophecy.

The idea of having patients forget about what happened during a procedure has merits in the eyes of some clinicians explaining in part their liking of drugs such as the sedative midazolam for its amnesic side effects. Their goal of easing patient's distressful memory is understandable; however, these care providers may be cautioned that medically induced amnesia does not necessarily prevent a patient from hearing derogatory or careless remarks while "under," nor does the drug prevent patients from suffering adverse consequences from such remarks while in recovery.[(1)] We recommend a non-pharmacological approach to guard against the patient having bad memories of the procedure—mainly by providing good ones.

Begin by making it your habit to avoid making negative suggestions (See chapter 8, "Avoiding Negative Suggestions,") and make it a point during induction to immunize the patient against negative suggestions (See chapter 12, "Hypnosis by

Script"). When you take these steps upfront, there should be no worry about a patient remembering the procedure unfavorably. In our experience, knowing that they have been able to help themselves through the worries and challenges of the procedures makes patients feel proud. When patients have a memory of their trance, it should be a good one. If on the other hand, a patient tells you upfront he or she just wants to be out and/or not remember anything, you can help them forget by suggesting, "and remember to forget, or forget to remember..." or "and only remember the pleasant aspects of this experience and what is needed to help you heal well and fast."

Time Distortion

Remembered or not, time in hypnosis goes by fast and easily. The patient in case 22.1, "A Short Nap," found it difficult to grasp that the time period that seemed to have been just long enough for a very short snooze, actually had taken 40 minutes. This speeded up time perception during hypnosis is common. A patient undergoing an MRI scan came out of the scanner room with a radiant smile, "You said 45 minutes to an hour! It seemed like 20 minutes, max. It was great." One might say time goes by fast, when one is having fun.

Reorientation

At the end of the patient's test or procedure, it is time to reorient the patient to his or her natural state of awareness. A common device is counting. Some hypnotists count upward from one to three or to five or to ten; others count from a high number down to one. If you use a count upward from one to three to induce hypnosis as suggested in the "Study Script 12.1," it makes sense to count backwards from three to one to reorient. The Study Script counting method allows you to also tell patients that whenever they wish to regain their state of relaxation, they can count forward from one to three: on *one*, looking up, on *two*, taking a breath in and slowly closing their eyes, and on *three* breathing out, relaxing their eyes, and focusing on a sensation of floating. When they want to regain their natural state of awareness, they just need to count backwards from three down to one: on *three* rolling their eyes up; on *two* taking a breath in; and on *one*, breathing out, opening up their eyes, and being fully alert and refreshed. This method is especially helpful for procedures where it is likely that patients are interrupted in their trance by actions of the personnel. It is also helpful for patients who want to be fully in control of everything and want to be able to adapt on their own when they want to be in trance and when not.

If you have chosen other inductions, you may use the following wording for reorientation from trance:

> "Your procedure (test) is completed now. You can come back now, easily gently and safely, and at your own pace. You can come back to this time, this day, and this place feeling better than you have in a long, long time. I will be counting to five, and when I say *five* you will come back to your full awareness once again. On the count of *one*, you are coming up higher and higher; on the count of *two*, a little further now; on the count of *three*, you are halfway there. On the count of *four*, your eyes feel as if they are splashed with cool, sparkling, spring water; and at the count of *five*, your eyes are fully open now, you are fully alert and refreshed now."

Time to Return to the Natural State of Awareness

Occasionally patients like it so much in their hypnotic trance that they want to stay a little longer. If they have to go to a recovery room, you can have them, while still in their trance, move from the procedure table to a gurney and have them continue their hypnotic journey as they are transported to the recovery room. It such cases it is important to alert the receiving recovery room team that the patient is in hypnosis and advise them what to do when it is time to re-alert the patient.

If the patient, however, needs to transfer to an area where appropriate reorientation cannot be guaranteed, or is ready go home, you must make sure that he or she is fully awake and re-alerted before leaving. In these instances, you can use time distortion to accelerate the re-alerting process. For example, you might say:

> "You can take all the clock time you need. And hours seem like minutes, and minutes become seconds...coming back now easily gently and safely...whenever you are ready you can open your eyes...you can now become fully alert to this time, to this day, and to this place. And with each breath you take you feel better and better, fully awake, refreshed and delighted."

If a patient is resistant to coming out of trance, don't panic. All patients eventually will come out of hypnosis. Sometimes you can use accelerators, such as asking the patients whether they can feel their full bladder and whether it is time to come back and go to the bathroom. There is an old saying that hypnosis will not work when either the patient or the hypnotist needs to go to the restroom—the subconscious imprint to control this urge is too strong.(1) Sometimes just reminding the patient about the happenings of the outside world does the trick.

JOURNAL ENTRY 22.1

Time to Go

Dr. Laser gave a smoking session class with a hypnotic group induction. Everyone of the particpants came back readily at the end of the session except for one man. The participants were leaving. Dr. Laser had collected her belongings. The cleaning people were coming in and out. Finally Dr. Laser said to the man: "Time to come back now. We have to lock the room. It is getting dark. The building will be closed and secured by the police, and a storm is coming and everybody is up and ready to leave." This did it. The man came back in an instant and both went on their way. ***Journal Notes, E. Laser***

Posthypnotic Suggestions for Recovery

Patients carry suggestions made in hypnosis into their daily life. You can take advantage of this phenomenon by making suggestions to help patients heal. In reorientation, you can include suggestions to the patient for a speedy recovery. You can specifically mention body functions that are pertinent to the type of procedure you did or that will counteract known side effects. You can say, "And when you awaken, all your vital organs will be working perfectly well. And, as each day goes by you will feel better and better. You will be able to urinate, to chew, to enjoy your food, to have regular bowel movements, to breathe easily—(or whatever is appropriate)."

You can also add suggestions for subsequent self-hypnosis and pain management in your reorientation and reinforce it with a repetition as follows:

> And now your procedure is completed. All your vital organs will be working perfectly well, and from now on anytime you might feel any discomfort you can go to the place you enjoy. All you have to do is close your eyes, breathe deeply, hold your thumb and forefinger together, and go to this wonderful place that you have enjoyed even during the height of your procedure and recovery.
>
> And you can come back now, easily, gently and safely and as slowly or quickly as you like. And, when you are ready to come back you can count yourself up from one to five and when you reach five you will be fully alert, fully awake, feeling

better than you have in a long, long time from these few brief minutes of hypnosis, taking all the time you need.

That's right, and every day in every way you are getting better and better—yes, better and better. All your vital organs will be working perfectly, and from now on anytime you might feel any discomfort you can go to the place you enjoy. All you have to do is close your eyes, breathe deeply, hold your thumb and forefinger together, and go to this wonderful place that you have enjoyed even during the height of your procedure and recovery. Come back to this time, to this date, to this place fully alert from these few brief minutes of hypnosis. Nowoooo.

The patient will do just that—he or she will come back. The patient will have benefited from having the option of using hypnosis during the procedure and will be feeling good about the experience and, typically, having less pain and fewer side effects than he or she might have had without hypnosis. You will be feeling good, too, knowing that you were able to help the patient help him- or herself through this challenge.

Key Points to Remember

- Some patients may not remember that they experienced a hypnotic trance, or what happened during the procedure.
- Remembered or not, time in hypnosis goes by fast and easily.
- At the end of the patient's test or procedure, it is time to reorient the patient to his or her natural state of awareness. A common device is to associate reorientation steps with numbers, which are counted up from or down to one.
- Occasionally patients like it so much in their hypnotic trance that they want to stay a little longer.
- If the patient needs to leave the area or go home, you must make sure that he or she is fully awake and re-alerted before leaving.

- Sometimes just reminding the patient about the happenings of the outside world is all that is needed to awake them from hypnosis.
- All patients eventually will come out of hypnosis.
- Patients carry suggestions made in hypnosis into their daily life. You can take advantage of this phenomenon by making posthypnotic suggestions for patients' future well being and healing and how they can return to a state of self-hypnosis.

Opportunities to Practice

- Decide whether you want to count up or down for inductions and reorientations and practice your reorientation sequence.
- Consider what posthypnotic suggestions would be particularly helpful for the patients in your practice.

Acknowledgments

The journey of this book would have never been possible without the encouragement and support of the many who have taught us, shared their wisdom generously, nudged us to get going, and been the pillars in our personal lives. We want to thank our brilliant editor Joan Lewis for blending our voices and keeping us on track gently and firmly, Donna Wolfe for being our expert reader, and John Jenkins III for his patience and creative genius in the graphic design of our book and cover.

We want to express our special thanks to:

Drs. Judy Illes and Michael Vannier, who insisted that we use rigorous scientific standards and seek federal funding to explore the efficacy of hypnosis in the procedure room.

Dr. David Spiegel for having always been there to support this project with graciousness and intellectual generosity particularly when new obstacles turned up and seemed insurmountable or frustrating.

The Department of Veterans Administration Affairs Medical Center (VAMC) Palo Alto and the University of Iowa Hospital and Clinics for providing the first educational grants to help explore the methodologies used in this book, and the National Institute of Health and the U.S. Army Materiel Command for supporting the prospective randomized studies, which established their efficacy.

The amazing teaching faculty of the New England and Chicago Societies of Clinical Hypnosis, the Society of Clinical and Experimental Hypnosis, and the American Society of Clinical Hypnosis.

The interventional radiology and research teams who have worked with us over the years, testing and refining what is found in this book, particularly Drs. Lauri Fick, Eric Benotsch, Olga Hatsiopoulou, Noami Halsey, Verena Stinshoff, Christine Schupp, Eva Kettenmann, Salomao Faintuch, and Gloria M. Salazar.

Drs. Susan Lugendorf, Henrietta Logan, and Kevin Berbaum; Brad Anderson, Donna Wolfe, and Debbie Philips for their unwavering support, professionalism, and friendship.

The men who each provided us individually anchor, love, and support: Joseph Lang, PhD for Elvira Lang; and members of her family and Steve Becker, MD for Eleanor Laser.

The patients for having volunteered to participate in the prospective randomized studies to enable the evidence-based practice of *Patient Sedation Without Medication*. They are the true heroes in this story.

Appendix of Hypnosis Scripts

The following are complete scripts and separate script elements, which you can use in your practice or adjust and combine to suit you particular needs. The chapter of this book in which each appears is indicted. If you would like script copies formatted to fit 8.5 x 11 paper, you may obtain full page files from the Hypnalgesics website at **www.hypnalgesics.com/script.**

Complete Scripts

Script 1.1 Experiencing Confidence

(Appears in chapter 1, "Building Confidence.")

Take a few slow breaths in and out. You may want to say to yourself with each breath in "strength;" and with each exhale imagine you blow out tension as you breathe out. You might notice how with each inhalation you take in more strength and confidence and with exhalation you let go of even more tension. You may want to do this a few times at your own rhythm, naturally and comfortably. And as you take a few moments to enjoy these liberating breaths, notice how breathing in this way makes you feel. If you hear sounds or noises in the room, just use these to deepen your experience. And use only the suggestions that are helpful for you.

Now, you can float to a time when everything just worked out well for you, one of those "magical" moments when everything just "clicked" and came together for you. It may have been a private moment or a public achievement, when something came true and through for you because you worked hard. You might have persevered and succeeded, or something just happened, something good, something good just by itself. Or when something you had learned came in very handy—one of these moments when you realize that you know how to meet the needs of the situation. And you say, "Yes! This is it!" and you fully experience the delight of this feeling. If you cannot think of such a personal experience like that right now, imagine what it might be like to have such an experience. Perhaps you have seen an experience like that in a movie, or have heard a story about someone having such an experience. Put yourself fully into that scenario.

Good. Now float further down into this magical moment in which everything just works out well. Enjoy this moment and savor the sights and sounds; wrap the feelings of achievement and delight around you.

You might even notice a color that permeates the scene. If so, you can make this "your color" and whenever—later in your work and life—you wish to regain this wonderful state of accomplishment, confidence, and peace, you may just want to think of this color. You may even want to keep at hand an object of "your" color to remind you how to enter that state of self-assurance whenever you need it, but just thinking of the color can be a signal in itself. Or there may be a sound or song in the air that can be your reminder of this moment, and just recalling this sound or song can transport you back to this state of strength whenever you wish or need to.

Alternatively, you can put thumb and forefinger together while immersed in the experience, and, hereafter, you can use this touching of the thumb and forefinger as a signal to bring to you this feeling of accomplishment, confidence, and peace that you are enjoying now. You can use one or more of these techniques whenever you desire or need to return to that confident state, even in the toughest of circumstances.

One more thing, your unconscious mind has been going through a process of allowing itself to assimilate and organize all the information that you needed into a format that your conscious mind could easily use at any time. Although you may not be fully conscious of what your unconscious mind has processed, bring that information with you as you slowly float back above yourself.

When you are ready to return to your natural state of awareness, slowly count backwards from three to one, as follows: On three, take a deep breath in. On two, let a breath out. On one, be fully awake, delighted, and proud to know how you can use your mind to relax, and how you can use your mind to help yourself and to help others.

Script 12.1 The Study Script

(Appears in chapter 12, "Hypnosis by Script.")

We want you to help us to help you to learn a concentration exercise to help you get through the procedure more comfortably. It can be a way to help your body be more comfortable through the procedure and also deal with any discomfort that may come up during the procedure. It is just a form of concentration, like getting so caught up in a movie or a good book that you forget you are watching a movie or reading a book.

Now you may be interested to learn how you can use your imagination to enter a state of focused attention and physical relaxation. If you hear sounds or noises in the room, just use these to deepen your experience. And use only the suggestions that are helpful for you. There are a lot of ways to relax, but here is one simple way:

On *one*, you can do one thing—look up.

On *two*, two things, slowly close your eyes and take a deep breath.

On *three*, three things, breathe out, relax your eyes, and let your body float.

Good. Just imagine your whole body floating, floating right through the table, with each breath deeper and easier. Right now imagine that you are floating somewhere safe and comfortable, in a bath, a lake, a hot tub, or just floating in space, with each breath deeper and easier. Just notice how with each breath you let a little more tension out of your body as you let your whole body float, safe and comfortable; each breath deeper and easier. Good, now with your eyes closed and remaining in this state of concentration, please describe for me how your body is feeling right now. Where do you imagine yourself being? What is it like? Can you smell the air? Can you see what is around you? Good. Now this is your safe and pleasant place to be and you can use it in a sense to play a trick on the doctors *(or this whole procedure).* Your body has to be here, but you don't. So just spend your time being somewhere you would rather be.

Now, if there is some discomfort, and there may be some with the procedure as they prepare you and insert the line, or as you feel the dye entering your body, there is no point in fighting it. You can admit it, but then transform that sensation. If you feel some discomfort, you might find it helpful to make that part of your body to feel warmer, as if you were in a bath. Or cooler—if that is more comfortable—as if you had ice or snow on that part of your body. This warmth and coolness becomes a protective filter between you and the pain.

If you have any discomfort right now, imagine that you are applying a hot pack or that you are putting snow or ice on it and see what it feels like. Develop the sense of warm or cool or delicious tingling numbness to filter the hurt out of the pain.

With each breath, breathe deeper and easier, your body is floating, filter the hurt out of the pain.

Now, again with your eyes closed and remaining in the state of concentration, describe what you are feeling right now.

(Option 1) ***If patient is at his or her safe and comfortable place—reinforce it. Say:***

What is it like now? What do you see around you? What are you doing?

(Option 2) ***If patient is in pain—address it. Say:***

The pain is there but see if you can add coolness or more warmth or make it lighter or make it heavier.

(Option 1) ***If patient is no longer in pain, say:***

Good. Continue to focus on those sensations.

(Option 2) ***If patient is still in pain, say:***

Focus on sensations in another part of your body. Now rub your fingertips together and notice all of the delicate sensations in your fingertips and see how much you can observe about what it feels like to rub your thumb and forefingers together. How do you feel now?

(Option 1) ***If patient is not in pain, say:***

Good. Continue to focus on these sensations.

(Option 2) ***If patient is still in pain, say:***

Now imagine yourself being at ______ (patient's safe place) where you said you felt relaxed and comfortable. What is it like now? What is the temperature? What do you see around you?

(Option 3) ***If patient states that he or she is worried—address it. Say:***

Okay, your main job right now is to help your body feel comfortable so we will talk about what is worrying you. But first, no matter what we discuss, concentrate on your body floating. So let's get the floating back into your body. Imagine that you are in this favorite spot and when you are ready let me know by nodding your head; and then we will talk about what is worrying you. But remember no matter what we discuss, concentrate on your body floating and feel safe and comfortable. So what is worrying you? *(Discuss)*

How do you feel now?

(Option 1) ***If patient is no longer worried, say:***

Good. Now continue to concentrate on your body floating, and feel safe and comfortable in your favorite place.

(Option 2) ***If patient is still worried, say:***

Okay, picture in your mind a screen like a movie screen, TV screen or a piece of clear blue sky. First you might see a pleasant scene on it. Now picture a large piece of blue screen divided in half. All right. Now on the left half, picture what you are worrying about on the screen. Now on the right half of the screen, picture what you will do about it, or what you would recommend someone else do about it. Keep your body floating. And if you are worrying about the outcome, okay admit it to yourself, but your body does not have to get uptight about it. You may, but your body does not have to.

Good. You know that whatever happens there is always something you can do. But for now just concentrate on keeping your body floating and feeling safe and comfortable.

From time to time throughout the procedure, say:

If you feel any sense of discomfort, you are welcome to let me know about it. You may use the filter to filter the hurt out of the pain, but by all means let me know and I will do what I can to help you with it as well. Whatever you do just keep your body floating and concentrate on being in the place where you feel safe and comfortable.

When the procedure is finished, say:

Okay, the procedure is completed now. We are going to formally leave this state of concentration by counting backwards from three to one. On *three* get ready, on *two* with your eyes closed roll up your eyes, and on *one* let your eyes open and take a deep breath and let it out. That will be the end of the formal exercise, but when you come out of it, you will still have the feeling of comfort that you felt during it. Ready, three, two, one.

If the patient opens the eyes, say:

Take a deep breath, and feel refreshed and proud about having helped yourself through this procedure.

If the patient hasn't followed, say:

Three—get ready. *Two* with your eyes closed, roll up your eyes. *One*—let your eyes open and take a deep breath, and feel refreshed and proud about having helped yourself through this procedure.

Script 16.1 The Floating Stone

(Appears in chapter 16, "Uses and Misuses of Trying.")

Become loose and comfortable; comfort is the key. It's just like you and I going on a brief vacation. You may hear outside noises, but they will only help you to deepen your own experience. And use only the suggestions that are helpful for you.

You can begin by looking up at a spot on the ceiling, high above your forehead. That's right. You may notice how your eyes begin to relax, and feel very heavy. There are very tiny little eyelid muscles in your eyelids, and they are very easy to control. Relax them completely to a point where they will not work. And when you are sure, and be sure in your own mind, and you have made the decision that they are completely relaxed to a point where they will not work, it is important to test and try to see that they will not work. Try now to open your eyes—but why bother. Okay, now stop trying.

Now you can send that relaxed feeling that you have in your eyelids throughout your entire face, your neck, feeling your jaw relaxing; your lips separating; and even your hair relaxing, too. Now allow this relaxation to spread throughout your whole body, from the top of your head to the tip of your toes.

Now, you can allow yourself to see the healing color of purple and all its glorious hues, or the color of your choice. And you can dive into this color, into all its delicious tones and shimmering lights, and feel wrapping all its gorgeous hues around you in a blanket of anesthesia and bliss, allowing your body to feel relaxed, calm, numb, courageous, and safe. You may feel numb just where it needs to be numb and for as long as it needs to be so. Relaxed, calm, numb, courageous, and safe. And this will be your mantra from now on as you begin to inhale. Breathe in to the count of four through your nostrils, pause into the gap, and exhale down through your nostrils all the way down and out to the count of eight. And continue this breathing through the entire time. In to the count of four, pause, and exhale through your nostrils all the way down and out continuing to say your words, your mantra: *relaxed, calm, numb, courageous, and safe.*

So now, we can begin to descend even deeper still. Go to a pleasant place, a beautiful safe place. A place of comfort and tranquility, a place of your choice. It might be on a mountain top with a creek, or home in your bed, or on a beach somewhere, or floating in the water of a lake or a pool, or even walking down a path. Wherever you find yourself, you can go there now, and you can begin to go down three deeper floors of hypnosis. And you can do this with your imagination and your imagination alone.

Perhaps you might enjoy seeing someone on the shore skipping a stone on the surface of the calm clear lake. As the stone ripples along, all worries and negative feelings that are not helpful to you ripple away. Then the stone comes to a place where it begins to float down. As you imagine the stone floating down to reach floor *A* you are floating to floor *A* of trance. And just as the stone freely floats down further, you descend along in your mind gently and safely to your floor *B* of trance. That's right. And when you are at floor *B* you can try to formulate the letter *B* but it is not possible. You cannot, no matter how hard you try, say the letter *B*. Try now. That's right. And as the stone begins to float down even further still, all the way down to the deepest level *C*, so can you allow yourself in your mind to go along down all the way to floor *C* of trance. Once again you can try to say, *"C"*, but no matter how hard you try, you cannot say the letter *C*. You can also try to pick up your leg *(or lift your hand or thumb or whatever—depending on the procedure)*, but you cannot. No matter how hard you try, you cannot raise your leg *(or lift your hand, etc.)*. This is a very deep level.

And, as you allow yourself to continue your breathing, in to the count of four, pause, into the gap, and exhale through your nostrils to the count of eight, down and out, you continue to repeat your words: *relaxed, calm, numb, courageous,* and *safe.*

And now, when you are ready to ascend again to your natural sate of awareness, you can float up from floor *C* to *B* and then to *A*. You can take with you the memory of only the pleasant things about this experience and the pride of knowing how you can help yourself so well. You can take this positive and pleasant feeling with you. You can count from one to five and with each count becoming more alert, more refreshed. One: getting ready.
Two: starting to open your eyes. Three: gently stretching. Four: further opening your eyes. And five: being fully alert, refreshed,

delighted, and proud of how you have been able help yourself through this procedure.

Script 17.2 Progressive Muscle Relaxation

(Appears in chapter 17, "Direct and Indirect Language.")

I would like to invite you to begin—either with your eyes open or closed—by allowing your body to relax and rest comfortably against the table. Now you may want to slowly take a breath in through your nose...hold...then exhale out through your mouth. At your own pace, you can take again a deep breath in through your nose...hold it...then exhale through your mouth.

Now, as you continue this deep, relaxing breathing, you may be surprised to notice how just the act of breathing alone can help your body to relax and feel more comfortable. You might be curious to find out how you can relax your body even more. You can do this by focusing on some of the smallest muscles in your body: the muscles in your eyes. Tighten those muscles as hard as you can and close the eyes as firmly as you can. You will know when these muscles are as tight as they can be, and then you can you enjoy the wonderful feeling of letting their tension go, having them become completely relaxed and limp. Or you may not even need to tighten them first, and can just send a delicious sensation of relaxation down into these tiny muscles. And the muscle of your right eye may relax first or the muscle of your left eye may relax fist, or both may relax together; or they already may be so relaxed that they wouldn't work even if you tried.

You might experience this feeling of relaxation as pleasant warmth, or you might see a calming white light. Now, allow this relaxing sensation to flow from your eyes, up into your eyebrows, and now up over the top of your head. And while you continue to breathe deeply and naturally, you may notice how with each breath the relaxation spreads...over the top of your head, down the back of your head, over your ears, and down into your neck. Let this pleasant and soothing sensation now cause your whole head and neck to become completely relaxed and at ease.

And you may focus now on your breath; with each breath you inhale, you inhale relaxation. And you will notice how with each breath you exhale, you exhale any tension and any discomfort and any stress that you might be feeling. Good. It is almost as if you can breath the tension right out of your body through the pores of your skin.

Now, allow the sensation to spread down your shoulders... down your arms and your hands, and right down to the tips of your fingers. Enjoy feeling how the relaxation spreads across your back, and down through your abdomen...into your legs, and down through your calves, to the tips of your toes. That's right. And if there's any place in your body that would like to feel even more relaxed than it already is notice its location without forcing or willing it. You can just take a very deep breath...hold this breath... and now exhale. This is called a *signal breath.* It can become your way of signaling your body to allow yourself to become even more fully relaxed and comfortable. When you take your signal breath, imagine that you are inhaling relaxation and comfort, and allow that breath to focus on the very spot of your body that you would like to feel even more relaxed. And now you can use your signal breath and inhale relaxation, and allow the exhaled breath to go right to that spot, and breathe any tension right out through the skin at that spot. You know when you will be ready to let relaxation and calm replace any feeling of tightness, discomfort, or tension; it may be now or in a few moments from now.

Now any time during the procedure that you would like to feel more relaxed and more comfortable, you can use your signal breath to breathe calming relaxation to that spot to help you feel completely at ease.

You may notice lots of noises around you during the procedure; people will be talking and moving, the equipment will make noises, and the lights will go on and off quite often. As you are aware of these things, just allow them to take you even deeper into a state of complete relaxation and comfort.

While the procedure is under way, you may have questions about what's going on around you. You know that you can remain in your fully relaxed state of calm, and still be able to ask whatever questions you would like. I will answer them for you, or I will find out the answers for you.

When the procedure is completed, or whenever you decide, you can return to your regular alert state by simply counting from one to three, either in your head or out loud. When you do this, you will find that even in your alert and fully attentive state you will continue to benefit from the calming sense of relaxation you now feel. And you can return to this place of calm whenever you like, by simply closing your eyes for a moment, counting back from three to one, and taking your signal breath, and feeling refreshed and fully alert.

Partial Scripts

Confusional Script

(Appears in chapter 14, "Confusional Inductions.")

You can go into a relaxed place at your own pace, you can relax deeply, and you can do this now, or in a moment from now. Everyone knows the importance of doing some homework. One never stops learning, so experience is a great teacher. There are lots of ways to get to a stoplight. When you first learn how to drive, while you think that it's important to stop, you might remember a time when you stepped on the gas to get there fast, and then you hurried up to stop.

Now, your eyes won't close until your inner mind gives you permission. That's great, and it's nice to know that you might remember back sometime when you enjoyed sinking your teeth into a nice juicy peach, or into a nice Mars bar. That's right, and even though Mars has a bar, there are many bars in Mars. Did you know that? Have you ever read about Mars, or maybe you saw it on Star Trek or Star Deck. Yes, that's the ticket to go there now, or you may go to another place of interest that you might enjoy. A person can be resourceful in so many ways, and there are a variety of ways to solve a problem. While I don't know what you do, or enjoy doing, and I don't know what you like to do best, but it's a fun idea to explore and go to a place of fun, of pleasant surroundings, and peace.

Wow, let's be on our way. And while we are going there, the other part of you is here getting repaired to really enjoy everything possible. Time flies when we are having fun, and one can spend time in a variety of ways. You can focus on making the best use of time, while your playful self enjoys it. You don't even have to listen to my voice because your unconscious mind will hear it clearly. There is nothing you have to do right now, nothing you have to think about or respond to. You don't even have to expect anything in particular.

Script 14.1 Confusion Induction

(Appears in chapter 14, "Confusional Inductions.")

You can go into a relaxed place at your own pace, you can relax deeply, and you can do this now, or in a moment from now.

Everyone knows the importance of doing some homework. One never stops learning, so experience is a great teacher.

There are lots of ways to get to a stoplight. When you first learn how to drive, while you think that it's important to stop, you might remember a time when you stepped on the gas to get there fast, and then you hurried up to stop.

Now, your eyes won't close until your inner mind gives you permission. Yes, that's right. And now, you can go down that bike path, riding down the trail, lowering down the hill, and you can go just as fast as your safety inner gauge allows you to go, and while the wind is blowing through your hair, and the sun is kissing your face, you can feel so free. And the constriction you might have felt, is leaving you, blowing in the breeze, and fading away in the air. And you know that that was a challenge, riding down that mountain, it is one thing to climb up, it's hard and it requires lots of work, and struggle, but all those past stifles, just enhanced your life up to now. And its good to know that while riding down this mountain, free as a bird, you can let go, yes let go, free of those past restrictions, that used to bind you and control you, so that now, while riding downhill on your bike, the limitless, unbound, open, released, feeling a new feeling of emancipation is wrapping you in a blanket of complete and utter energy. You no longer have to be chained and leashed to respond in the old ways, new and inviting behavior is taking charge. And you don't even have to listen to my voice, because you're unconscious mind will hear it clearly. There is nothing you have to do right now, nothing you have to think about or respond to. You don't even have to expect anything in particular. And, time flies when we are having fun. And one can spend time in a variety of ways. You can focus on making the best use of time, while your playful self enjoys it.

Script 14.2 Conscious-Unconscious Dissociation Induction

(Appears in chapter 14, "Confusional Inductions.")

Your conscious mind might be listening to my voice while your unconscious mind is very busy attending to important matters; while your conscious mind may not fully trust hypnosis, your unconscious mind is concerned with what is safe; perhaps your conscious mind may be doubtful, but your unconscious mind can find security, because, it thinks in a broader scope; your conscious mind may be cautious and take precaution while your unconscious mind can often select the depth of trance it decides to go; and your conscious mind often knows and watches, while your unconscious mind protects and guides you; as your conscious mind may hear my words, while your unconscious mind can allow you to deepen your trance, and does hear and knows; while your conscious mind wonders how to, your unconscious mind already knows and discovers how.

Internal Dialogue

(Appears in chapter 17, "Direct and Indirect Language.")

Your eyes won't close until your inner mind gives you permission. As you are lying here, you might feel a little tingling and you might find one part of your body feeling different. As you are continuing to listen to my voice, I've noticed that your breathing has slowed a bit, and down you can float, letting go. You feel like you might be floating on a cloud or on a magic carpet, flying over a place you might like to visit again or that you have always wanted to visit. And now... (validate what you see, responding to the patient in reference to what you notice, such as "that you are breathing more slowly," or "have your hand relaxed against your side,") and as you travel to your destination, you may be experiencing some numbness in your hand or somewhere in your body and that's all right, and your eyes might want to close down and seal shut. You can develop numbness in your hand as you drop it into ice cold water, and you can move it to another place and transfer the numbness to your face and your tooth, but that tooth can stay in trance even though you can sink into the bed, dreaming of a ride on a bus to a beautiful place. Yes, that's good. I don't know where you are, but I have noticed that you might be going deep down into a deep relaxed place, and that's all right. You can go into your unconscious mind...go there now, and into the most wonderful opportunity to heal, have fun, and mend. There is no use waiting any longer. It is there now, so you can go way down, deeper and deeper, into the most relaxed feeling you ever had. There's no sense in holding you back. Things occur in their own way and time. As you allow yourself to reach your goal, it's important to slide down into trance and go inside yourself. You can go into a relaxed place at your own pace. You can relax deeply, and you can do this now, or in a moment from now.

Parts Model for Distress Management

(Appears in chapter 19, "Managing Anxiety and Distress.")

Go to the part that is creating the feeling of being scared (or that is giving you this feeling). Take a body scan and you will feel the part signal you—you might feel a flutter or a squeeze or heaviness or something similar, and when you feel the feeling in your body; let us know where it is. *(Either a nod of the head or an ideomotor signal will indicate it.)* Okay, thank you. Ask the part to come forward so that you can see it in front of you. You can hold it in your hands or look at it. Now give the part a voice. And now, ask the part what it is that it wants for you? It has good intentions and it will tell you. Ask the part if it would enjoy helping you do another job? Tell the part you appreciate its positive intention and loyalty over the years. It never even asked for a raise. Now we need the part's help to protect you in this new experience during your procedure. Can we count on the part to help? Thank the part again. Just let yourself relax now. The part will help you stay well.

Script 19.1 The Red Balloon

(Appears in chapter 19, "Managing Anxiety and Distress.")

Imagine a meadow, filled with gorgeous colorful flowers, blue, yellow, red, and lavender, all of its vibrancy shone far into the distance. You are lured to this gorgeous, glorious place, and as you walk closer and closer, you see a huge red balloon. As you continue to come closer, you realize that the red balloon is tied to a huge basket and has another basket within. And now, you see that the outer basket is weighted down by sandbags. You remove the inner basket and hear within yourself, that you are to place all your worries, self doubts, fears, complaints, disenchantments, and all other negative beliefs into the inner basket. You have all the time you need. As you face the basket, you soon place every feeling that you want to unload, into the container. As you do, you begin to feel less constraint and burdened. Now, imagine putting the filled inner basket back into the outer basket, and then imagine your hands untying the ropes that hold the outer basket to the weights, and as each rope is untied, a sandbag falls to the ground. As the sandbags fall, you now have the power to let go, to release, and unburden your inner self. You have now gained enjoyment in life, and begin a new day. As the red balloon lifts the container away, you can actually feel the burdens of self-doubt, anxieties, fears, worries, and all negative beliefs, lifted from your shoulders. As the balloon continues to raise high in the sky, finally into the universe, you can only see a faint dot, a tiny hue of red that fades away in the sunset. From now on, you can recreate this image from your memory, and continue to enjoy life with a new positive approach feeling relieved and refreshed.

Reorientation Excerpt

(Appears in chapter 22, "Reorientation.")

"Your procedure (test) is completed now. You can come back now, easily gently and safely, and at your own pace. You can come back to this time, this day, and this place feeling better than you have in a long, long time. I will be counting to five, and when I say *five* you will come back to your full awareness once again. On the count of *one*, you are coming up higher and higher; on the count of *two*, a little further now; on the count of *three*, you are halfway there. On the count of *four*, your eyes feel as if they are splashed with cool, sparkling, spring water; and at the count of *five*, your eyes are fully open now, you are fully alert and refreshed now."

Reorientation: Time Distortion to Accelerate the Re-alerting Process

(Appears in chapter 22, "Reorientation.")

"You can take all the clock time you need. And hours seem like minutes, and minutes become seconds...coming back now easily gently and safely...whenever you are ready you can open your eyes...you can now become fully alert to this time, to this day, and to this place. And with each breath you take you feel better and better, fully awake, refreshed and delighted."

Reorientation: Suggestions For Subsequent Self-Hypnosis and Pain Management

(Appears in chapter 22, "Reorientation.")

And now your procedure is completed all your vital organs will be working perfectly well, and from now on anytime you might feel any discomfort you can go to the place you enjoy. All you have to do is close your eyes, breathe deeply, hold your thumb and forefinger together, and go to this wonderful place that you have enjoyed even during the height of your procedure and recovery.

And you can come back now, easily, gently and safely and as slowly or quickly, as you like. And, when you are ready to come back you can count yourself up from one to five and when you reach five you will be fully alert, fully awake, feeling better than you have in a long, long time from these few brief minutes of hypnosis, taking all the time you need.

That's right, and every day in every way you are getting better and better—yes, better and better. All your vital organs will be working perfectly, and from now on anytime you might feel any discomfort you can go to the place you enjoy. All you have to do is close your eyes, breathe deeply, hold your thumb and forefinger together, and go to this wonderful place that you have enjoyed even during the height of your procedure and recovery. Come back to this time, to this date, to this place fully alert from these few brief minutes of hypnosis. Nowoooo.

References

Chapter 1

1. Moss Kanter, Rosabeth. 2004. *How winning streaks & losing streaks begin and end.* New York: Crown Business.
2. Neumann, Roland, and Fritz Strack. 2000. "Mood contagion": The automatic transfer of mood between persons. *Journal of Personality and Social Psychology* 79:211-233.
3. Lang, Elvira V., Eric G. Benotsch, Lauri J. Fick, Susan Lutgendorf, Michael L. Berbaum, Kevin S. Berbaum, Henrietta Logan, and David Spiegel. 2000. Adjunctive non-pharmacologic analgesia for invasive medical procedures: A randomized trial. *Lancet* 355:1486-1490.
4. Lang, Elvira V., Kevin S. Berbaum, Salomao Faintuch, Olga Hatsiopoulou, Noami Halsey, Xinyu Li, Michael L. Berbaum, Eleanor Laser, and Janet Baum. 2006. Adjunctive self-hypnotic relaxation for outpatient medical procedures: A prospective randomized trial with women undergoing large core breast biopsy. *Pain* 126:155-164.
5. Lang, Elvira V., Kevin S. Berbaum, Stephen Pauker, Salomao Faintuch, Gloria Maria Salazar, Susan K. Lutgendorf, Eleanor Laser, Henrietta Logan, and David Spiegel. 2008. Beneficial effects of hypnosis and adverse effects of empathic attention during percutaneous tumor treatment: When being nice does not suffice. *Journal of Vascular and Interventional Radiology* 19:897-905.

Chapter 2

1. Pederson, Cort A., 2004. Biological aspects of social bonding and the roots of human violence. *Annals of the New York Academy of Sciences* 1036:106-127.
2. Mobbs, Dean, Predrag Petrovic, Jennifer L. Marchant, Demis Hassabis, Nikolaus Weiskopf, Ben Seymour, Raymond J. Dolan, and Christopher D. Frith. 2007. When fear is near: Threat imminence elicits prefrontal-periaqueductal gray shifts in humans. *Science* 317:1079-1083.
3. Adams, Leslie, and David Zuckerman. 1991. The effect of lighting conditions on personal space requirements. *The Journal of General Psychology* 118:335-341.
4. Geden, Elizabeth A., and Ann V. Begeman. 1981. Personal space preferences of hospitalized adults. *Research in Nursing & Health* 2:237-241.
5. Williams, Lawrence E., and John A. Bargh. 2008. Keeping one's distance: The influence of spatial distance cues on affect and evaluation. *Psychological Science* 19:302-308.

Chapter 3

1. Iacoboni, Marco. 2009. Imitation, empathy, and mirror neurons. *Annual Review of Psychology* 60:653-670.
2. Meltzoff, Andrew N., and Jean Decety. 2003. What imitation tells us about social cognition: A rapprochement between developmental psychology and cognitive neuroscience. *Philosophical Transactions of the Royal Society London* B 358:491-500.
3. di Pellegrino, G., L. Fadiga, L. Fogassi, V. Gallese, and Giacomo Rizzolatti. 1992. Understanding motor events: A neurophysiological study. *Experimental Brain Research* 91:176-180.
4. Kohler, Evelyne, Christian Keysers, M. Alessandra Umilta, Leonardo Fogassi, Vittorio Gallese, and Giacomo Rizzolati. 2002. Hearing sounds, understanding actions: Action representation in mirror neurons. *Science* 297:846-848.
5. Paukner, Annika, James R. Anderson, Eleonora Borelli, Elisabetta Viosalberghi, and Pier F. Ferrari. 2005. Macaques (Macaca nemestrina) recognize when they are being imitated. *Biology Letters* 1:219-222.
6. Chartrand, Tanya L., and John A. van Bargh. 1999. The chameleon effect: The perception-behavior link and social interaction. *Journal of Personality and Social Psychology* 76:893-910.
7. van Baaren, Rick B., William Maddux, W., and Tanya L. Chartrand. 2003. It takes two to mimic: Behavioral consequences of self-construals. *Journal of Personality and Social Psychology* 94:1093-1102.
8. Bernieri, Frank J., Janet Davis, M., John S. Gillis, and Jon E. Grahe. 1996. Dyad rapport and the accuracy of its judgment across situations: A lens model analysis. *Journal of Personality and Social Psychology* 71:110-129.

Chapter 4

1. Miles, Lyndon K., Louise K. Nind, and C. Neil Macrae. 2009. The rhythm of rapport: Interpersonal synchrony and social perception. *Journal of Experimental Social Psychology* 45:585-589.
2. van Baaren, Rick B., William Maddux, W., and Tanya L. Chartrand. 2003. It takes two to mimic: Behavioral consequences of self-construals. *Journal of Personality and Social Psychology* 94:1093-1102.

Chapter 5

1. Dilts, Robert, John Grinder, Richard Bandler, and Judith DeLozier. 1980. *Neurolinguistic programming. Volume 1: The study of subjective experience.* Cupertino, CA: Meta Publications.
2. Weitzenhofer, Andre M. 1989. Ericksonian hypnotism: The Bandler/Grinder interpretation. In *The practice of hypnotism.* New York: John Wiley & Sons.

Chapter 6

1. Dilts, Robert, John Grinder, Richard Bandler, and Judith DeLozier. 1980. *Neurolinguistic programming. Volume 1: The study of subjective experience.* Cupertino, CA: Meta Publications.
2. Gladwell, Malcolm. 2002. *The naked face. Can you read people's thoughts just by looking at them?:* The New Yorker, August 5. http://www.gladwell.com/ 2002/2002_08_05_a_face.htm.
3. Frischen, Alexandra, Andrew P. Bayliss, and Steven P. Tipper. 2007. Gaze cueing of attention: Visual attention, social cognition, and individual differences. *Psychological Bulletin* 133:694-724.
4. Calder, Andrew J., Andrew D. Lawrence, Jill Keane, Sophie K. Scott, Adrian M. Owen, Ingrid Christoffels, and Andrew W. Young. 2002. Reading the mind from eye gaze. *Neuropsychologia* 40:1129-1138.

Chapter 7

1. Guéguen, Nicolas, Céline Jacob, and Gaélle Boulbry. 2007. The effect of touch on compliance with a restaurant's employee suggestion. *Hospitality Management* 26:1019-1023.
2. Erceau, Damien, and Nicolas Guéguen. 2007. Tactile contact and evaluation of the toucher. *The Journal of Social Psychology* 147:441-444.
3. Drescher, Vincent M., Horsley Gantt, and William E. Whitehead. 1980. Heart rate response to touch. *Psychosomatic Medicine* 42:559-565.
4. Chapell, M. S., W. Beltran, M. Santanello, M. Takahashi, S. R. Bantom, and J. S. Donovan. 1999. Men and women holding hands: II. Whose hand is uppermost? *Perceptual and Motor Skills* 89:537-549.
5. Estabrooks, Carole A., and Janice Morse, M. 1992. Towards a theory of touch: the touching process and acquiring a touching style. *Journal of Advanced Nursing* 17:448-456.
6. Lecron, Leslie M. 1964. *Self-hypnotism; The technique and its use in daily living.* Englewood Cliffs, NJ: Prentice-Hall, Inc.
7. Cheek, David B. 1994. *Hypnosis: The application of ideomotor signals.* Needham Heights, MA: Allyn and Bacon: A Division of Paramount Publishing.

Chapter 8

1. Lang, Elvira V., Kevin S. Berbaum, and Susan K. Lutgendorf. 2009. Large-core breast biopsy: Abnormal salivary cortisol profiles associated with uncertainty of diagnosis. *Radiology* 250:631-637.
2. Silvestri, Antonello, Pasquale Galetta, Elena C. Cerquetani, Giuseppe Marazzi, Roberto Patrizi, Massimo Fini, and Giuseppe M. C. Rosano. 2003. Report of erectile dysfunction after therapy with beta-blockers is related to patient knowledge of side effects and is reversed by placebo. *European Heart Journal* 24:1928-1932.

3. Ewin, Dabney M., and Bruce N. Eimer. 2006. *Ideomotor signals for rapid hypnoanalysis.* Springfield, IL: Charles C. Thomas Publishers.

4. Bayer, Timothy L., John H. Coverdale, Elizabeth Chiang, and Mark Bangs. 1998. The role of prior pain experience and expectancy in psychologically and physically induced pain. *Pain* 74:327-331.

5. Spiegel, Herbert. 1997. Nocebo: The power of suggestibility. *Preventive Medicine* 26:616-621.

6. Lang, Elvira V., Olga Hatsiopoulou, Timo Koch, Susan Lutgendorf, Eva Kettenmann, Henrietta Logan, and Ted J. Kaptchuk. 2005. Can words hurt? Patient-provider interactions during invasive medical procedures. *Pain* 114:303-309.

7. Lang, Elvira V., Kevin S. Berbaum, Salomao Faintuch, Olga Hatsiopoulou, Noami Halsey, Xinyu Li, Michael L. Berbaum, Eleanor Laser, and Janet Baum. 2006. Adjunctive self-hypnotic relaxation for outpatient medical procedures: A prospective randomized trial with women undergoing large core breast biopsy. *Pain* 126:155-164.

Chapter 9

1. Karasek, R. A. 1979. Job demands, job decision latitude and mental strain: Implications for job redesign. *Administrative Science Quarterly* 24:285-308.

2. deLange, Annet H., Toon W. Taris, Irene L. D. Houtman, Michiel A. J. Kompier, and Paulien M. Bongers. 2003. "The very best of the millenium": Longitudinal research and the Demand-Control-(Support) Model. *Journal of Occupational Health Psychology* 8:282-305.

3. van der Doef, Margot, and Stan Maes. 1999. The Job-Demand-Control (-Support) Model of psychological well-being; A review of 20 years of empirical research. *Work & Stress* 13:87-114.

4. Breier, A., M. Albus, D. Pickar, T. P. Zahn, O. M. Wolkowitz, and S. M. Paul. 1987. Controllable and uncontrollable stress in humans: Alteration in mood and neuroendocrine and psychophysiological function. *American Journal of Psychiatry* 144:1419-1425.

5. Staub, Ervin, Bernhard Tursky, and Gary E. Schwartz. 1971. Self-control and predictability: Their effects on reaction to aversive stimulation. *Journal of Personality and Social Psychology* 18:157-162.

6. Amat, J., M. V. Baratta, E. Paul, S. T. Bland, L. R. Watkins, and S. F. Maier. 2005. Medial prefrontal cortex determines how stressor controllability affects behavior and dorsal raphe nucleus. *Nature Neuroscience* 8:365-371.

7. Anderson, K., and F. Masur. 1983. Psychological preparation for invasive medical and dental procedures. *Journal of Behavioral Medicine* 6:1-40.

8. Like, Robert, and Stephen J. Zyzanski. 1987. Patient satisfaction with the clinical encounter: Social psychological determinants *Social Science & Medicine* 4:351-357.

9. Lang, Elvira V., Susan Lutgendorf, Henrietta Logan, Eric G. Benotsch, Eleanor Laser, and David Spiegel. 1999. Nonpharmacologic analgesia and anxiolysis for interventional radiological procedures. *Seminars in Interventional Radiology* 16:113-123.

Chapter 10

1. Dinkmeyer, Don, and Rudolf Dreikurs. 2000. *Encouraging children to learn.* Philadelphia, PA: Psychology Press, Brunner-Routledge.
2. Henderlong, Jennifer, and Mark P. Lepper. 2002. The effects of praise on children's intrinisc motivation: A review and synthesis. *Psychological Bulletin* 128:774-795.
3. Kohn, Alfie. 1993. *Punished by rewards: The trouble with gold stars, incentive plans, A's, praise, and other bribes.* New York: Houghton Mifflin.
4. Kanouse, D. E., P. Gumpert, and D. Canavan-Gumbert. 1981. The semantics of praise. In *New directions in attribution research,* edited by J. H. Harvey, W. Ickes and R. F. Kidd. Hillsdale, NJ: Erlbaum.

Chapter 11

1. Lang, Elvira V., Eric G. Benotsch, Lauri J. Fick, Susan Lutgendorf, Michael L. Berbaum, Kevin S. Berbaum, Henrietta Logan, and David Spiegel. 2000. Adjunctive non-pharmacologic analgesia for invasive medical procedures: A randomized trial. *Lancet* 355: 1486-1490.
2. Lang, Elvira V., Kevin S. Berbaum, Stephen Pauker, Salomao Faintuch, Gloria Maria Salazar, Susan K. Lutgendorf, Eleanor Laser, Henrietta Logan, and David Spiegel. 2008. Beneficial effects of hypnosis and adverse effects of empathic attention during percutaneous tumor treatment: When being nice does not suffice. *Journal of Vascular and Interventional Radiology* 19:897-905.
3. Spiegel, David. 1989. Uses and abuses of hypnosis. *Integrative Psychiatry* 6:211-222.
4. Spiegel, Herbert, and David Spiegel. 1978. *Trance and treatment: Clinical uses of hypnosis.* New York: Basic Books.
5. Ewin, Dabney M., and Bruce N. Eimer. 2006. *Ideomotor signals for rapid hypnoanalysis.* Springfield, IL: Charles C. Thomas Publishers.
6. Temes, Roberta. 2000. *The complete idiot's guide to hypnosis.* New York: Alpha Books, Penguin Group.
7. Barabasz, Arreed F. 2005. Wither spontaneous hypnosis: A critical issue for practitioners and researchers. *American Journal of Clinical Hypnosis* 48:2-3.
8. US Attorneys. 288 *Admissibility at trial, USAM Title 9 Criminal Resource Manual.* http://www.usdoj.gov/usao/eousa/foia_reading_room/usam/title9/crm00288.htm.

Chapter 12

1. Lang, Elvira V., Kevin S. Berbaum, Stephen Pauker, Salomao Faintuch, Gloria Maria Salazar, Susan K. Lutgendorf, Eleanor Laser, Henrietta Logan, and David Spiegel. 2008. Beneficial effects of hypnosis and adverse effects of empathic attention during percutaneous tumor treatment: When being nice does not suffice. *Journal of Vascular and Interventional Radiology* 19:897-905.
2. Blankfield, Robert P. 1991. Suggestion, relaxation, and hypnosis as adjuncts in the care of surgery patients: A review of the literature. *American Journal of Clinical Hypnosis* 33:172-186.
3. Spiegel, Herbert, and David Spiegel. 1978. *Trance and treatment: Clinical uses of hypnosis.* New York: Basic Books.

Chapter 13

1. Sparks, Laurance. 1962. *Self-hypnosis. A conditioned response technique.* New York: Wilshire Book Company, Grune & Stratton.
2. Page, Roger A., George W. Handley, and J. C. Carey. 2002. Can devices facilitate a hypnotic induction? *American Journal of Clincial Hypnosis* 45:137-141.
3. Gardner, G. Gail, and Karen Olness. 1981. *Hypnosis and hypnotherapy with children.* Orlando, FL: Grune & Stratton, Inc.
4. Spiegel, Herbert. 2007. The neural trance: A new look at hypnosis. *International Journal of Clinical and Experimental Hypnosis* 55:387-410.
5. Lee, Jun-Seok, David Spiegel, Sae-Byul Kim, Jang-Han Lee, Sun-Il Kim, Byung-Hwan Yang, Joon-Ho Choi, Yong-Chul Kho, and Jung-Hyun Nam. 2007. Fractal analysis of EEG in hypnosis and its relationship with hypnotizability. *International Journal of Clinical and Experimental Hypnosis* 55:14-31.
6. Spiegel, Herbert, and David Spiegel. 1978. *Trance and treatment: Clinical uses of hypnosis.* New York: Basic Books.

Chapter 14

1. Erickson, Milton H. 1980. *The collected papers of Milton Erickson. Volume 1. The nature of hypnosis and suggestions. Edited by Ernest L. Rossi.* New York: Irvington Publishers.
2. Hammond, C. Corydon. 1990. Formulating hypnotic and posthypnotic suggestions. In *Hypnotic suggestions and metaphors. An American Society of Clinical Hypnosis Book,* edited by C. C. Hammond. New York, London: W. W. Norton & Company.

Chapter 15

1. Lang, Elvira V., Cayte Ward, and Eleanor Laser. 2009. Effect of team training on patients' ability to complete MRI examinations. *Academic Radiology* In press.

2. Ewin, Dabney M., and Bruce N. Eimer. 2006. *Ideomotor signals for rapid hypnoanalysis.* Springfield, IL: Charles C. Thomas Publishers.

3. Weitzenhofer, Andre M. 1989. Ericksonian hypnotism: The Bandler/Grinder interpretation. In *The practice of hypnotism.* New York: John Wiley & Sons.

4. LeCron, Leslie M. 1954. A hypnotic technique for uncovering unconscious material. *Journal of Clinical and Experimental Hypnosis* 2:76-79.

5. Cheek, David B., and Leslie M. LeCron. 1968. *Clinical hypnotherapy.* New York: Grune & Stratton.

6. Rossi, Ernest L., and David B. Cheek. 1988. *Mind-body therapy. Methods of ideodynamic healing in hypnosis.* New York: W. W. Norton.

Chapter 16

1. Weitzenhofer, Andre M. 1989. *The practice of hypnotism. Volume 2. Applications of traditional and semi-traditional hypnotism. Non-traditional hypnotism.* Edited by I. B. Weiner, *Series on personality processes.* New York: John Wiley & Sons.

2. Hammond, C. Corydon. 1990. Formulating hypnotic and posthypnotic suggestions. In *Hypnotic suggestions and metaphors. An American Society of Clinical Hypnosis Book.,* edited by C. C. Hammond. New York, London: W. W. Norton & Company.

Chapter 17

1. Hammond, C. Corydon. 1984. Myths about Erickson and Ericksonian hypnosis. *American Journal of Clinical Hypnosis* 26:236-245.

2. ———. 1990. Formulating hypnotic and posthypnotic suggestions. In *Hypnotic suggestions and metaphors. An American Society of Clinical Hypnosis Book,* edited by C. C. Hammond. New York, London: W. W. Norton & Company.

Chapter 18

1. Lang, Elvira V., Cayte Ward, and Eleanor Laser. 2009. Effect of team training on patients' ability to complete MRI examinations. *Academic Radiology* In press.

2. Anonymous. 2001. Court victory for hypnosis woman. *BBC News UK 25 May.* http://news.bbc.co.uk/2/hi/uk_news/1352057.stm.

3. Fick, Lauri J., Elvira V. Lang, Henrietta L. Logan, Susan Lutgendorf, and Eric G. Benotsch. 1999. Imagery content during nonpharmacologic analgesia in the procedure suite: Where your patients would rather be. *Academic Radiology* 6:457-463.

Chapter 19

1. Schupp, Christine, Kevin S. Berbaum, Michael L. Berbaum, and Elvira V. Lang. 2005. Pain and anxiety during interventional radiological

procedures. Effect of patients' state anxiety at baseline and modulation by nonpharmacologic analgesia adjuncts *Journal of Vascular and Interventional Radiology* 16:1585-1592.

2. Daitch, Carolyn. 2007. *Affect regulation toolbox.* New York: W. W. Norton & Company.
3. Watkins, Helen H. 1993. Ego-state therapy: An overview. *American Journal of Clinical Hypnosis* 35:242-240.
4. Thomson, Linda. 2005. *Harry the Hypno-potamus. Metaphorical tales for the treatment of children.* Carmarthen, Wales, UK: Crown House Publishing Limited.Chapter 20.

Chapter 20

1. De Pascalis, Vilfredo, Immacolata Cacace, and Francesca Massicolle. 2008. Focused analgesia in waking and hypnosis: Effects on pain, memory, and somatosensory event-related potentials. *Pain* 134:197-208.
2. Rainville, Pierre, Gary H. Duncan, D. D. Price, B. Carrier, and M. Catherine Bushnell. 1997. Pain affect encoded in human anterior cingulate but not somatosensory cortex. *Science* 277:968-971.
3. Hofbauer, Robert K., Pierre Rainville, Gary H. Duncan, and M. Catherine Bushnell. 2001. Cortical representation of the sensory dimension of pain. *Journal of Neurophysiology* 86:402-411.
4. Schupp, Christine, Kevin S. Berbaum, Michael L. Berbaum, and Elvira V. Lang. 2005. Pain and anxiety during interventional radiological procedures. Effect of patients' state anxiety at baseline and modulation by nonpharmacologic analgesia adjuncts *Journal of Vascular and Interventional Radiology* 16:1585-1592.
5. Lang, Elvira V., Kevin S. Berbaum, Stephen Pauker, Salomao Faintuch, Gloria Maria Salazar, Susan K. Lutgendorf, Eleanor Laser, Henrietta Logan, and David Spiegel. 2008. Beneficial effects of hypnosis and adverse effects of empathic attention during percutaneous tumor treatment: When being nice does not suffice. *Journal of Vascular and Interventional Radiology* 19:897-905.
6. Lang, Elvira V., Kevin S. Berbaum, Salomao Faintuch, Olga Hatsiopoulou, Noami Halsey, Xinyu Li, Michael L. Berbaum, Eleanor Laser, and Janet Baum. 2006. Adjunctive self-hypnotic relaxation for outpatient medical procedures: A prospective randomized trial with women undergoing large core breast biopsy. *Pain* 126:155-164.
7. Lang, Elvira V., Eric G. Benotsch, Lauri J. Fick, Susan Lutgendorf, Michael L. Berbaum, Kevin S. Berbaum, Henrietta Logan, and David Spiegel. 2000. Adjunctive non-pharmacologic analgesia for invasive medical procedures: A randomized trial. *Lancet* 355:1486-1490.
8. Ewin, Dabney M., and Bruce N. Eimer. 2006. *Ideomotor signals for rapid hypnoanalysis.* Springfield, IL: Charles C. Thomas Publishers.

9. Bayer, Timothy L., John H. Coverdale, Elizabeth Chiang, and Mark Bangs. 1998. The role of prior pain experience and expectancy in psychologically and physically induced pain. *Pain* 74:327-331.

10. Hammond, C. Corydon. 2008. Hypnosis as sole anesthesia for major surgeries: Historical & contemporary perspectives. *American Journal of Clinical Hypnosis* 51:101-121.

11. Erickson III, James C. 1994. The use of hypnosis in anesthesia: A master class commentary. *International Journal of Clinical and Experimental Hypnosis* 42:8-12.

12. Spiegel, Herbert, and David Spiegel. 1978. *Trance and treatment: Clinical uses of hypnosis.* New York: Basic Books.

13. Montgomery, Guy H., Daniel David, Gary Winkel, Jeffrey H. Silverstein, and Dana H. Bovberg. 2002. The effectiveness of adjunctive hypnosis with surgical patients: A meta-analysis. *Anesthesia and Analgesia* 94:1639-1645.

14. Greenleaf, Marcia. 2008. In memoriam of Dr. Selig Finkelstein (1916-2008). *American Journal of Clinical Hypnosis* 51:99-100.

Chapter 21

1. Lang, Elvira V., Eric G. Benotsch, Lauri J. Fick, Susan Lutgendorf, Michael L. Berbaum, Kevin S. Berbaum, Henrietta Logan, and David Spiegel. 2000. Adjunctive non-pharmacologic analgesia for invasive medical procedures: A randomized trial. *Lancet* 355: 1486-1490.

2. Lang, Elvira V., Kevin S. Berbaum, Stephen Pauker, Salomao Faintuch, Gloria Maria Salazar, Susan K. Lutgendorf, Eleanor Laser, Henrietta Logan, and David Spiegel. 2008. Beneficial effects of hypnosis and adverse effects of empathic attention during percutaneous tumor treatment: When being nice does not suffice. *Journal of Vascular and Interventional Radiology* 19:897-905.

3. Zachariae, Robert, and Peter Bjerring. 1994. Laser-induced pain-related brain potentials and sensory pain ratings in high and low hypnotizable subjects during hypnotic suggestions of relaxation, dissociated imagery, focused analgesia, and placebo. *International Journal of Clinical and Experimental Hypnosis* 42:56-80.

4. DeBenedittis, Giuseppe, Mario Cigada, Anna Bianchi, Maria Gabriella Signorini, and Sergio Cerutti. 1994. Autonomic changes during hypnosis: A heart rate variability power spectrum analysis as a marker of sympathico-vagal balance. *International Journal of Clinical and Experimental Hypnosis* 42:140-152.

5. Hippel, C. V., G. Hole, and Wolfgang P. Kaschka. 2001. Autonomic profile under hypnosis as assessed by heart rate variability and spectral analysis. *Pharmacopsychiatry* 34:111-113.

6. Zachariae, Robert, Michael M. Jorgenson, Peter Bjerring, and Gunner Svendsen. 2000. Autonomic and psychological responses to an acute psychological stressor and relaxation: The influence of hypnotizability and absorption. *International Journal of Clinical and Experimental Hypnosis* 48:388-403.

7. Anderson, Jeffrey L., and Benjamin D. Horne. 2005. Nonlinear heart rate variability. *Journal of Cardiovascular Electrophysiology* 16:21-23.

8. Stein, Phyllis, Peter P. Domitrovich, Heikki V. Huikuri, Robert E. Kleiger, and for the CAST Investigators. 2005. Traditional and nonlinear heart rate variability are each independently associated with mortality after myocardial infarction. *Journal of Cardiovascular Electrophysiology* 16:13-20.

Chapter 22

1. Ewin, Dabney M., and Bruce N. Eimer. 2006. *Ideomotor signals for rapid hypnoanalysis.* Springfield, IL: Charles C. Thomas Publishers.

2. De Pascalis, Vilfredo, Immacolata Cacace, and Francesca Massicolle. 2008. Focused analgesia in waking and hypnosis: Effects on pain, memory, and somatosensory event-related potentials. *Pain* 134: 197-208.

Index

D

I

J

K

L

R

S

T

U

V

W

Elvira Lang

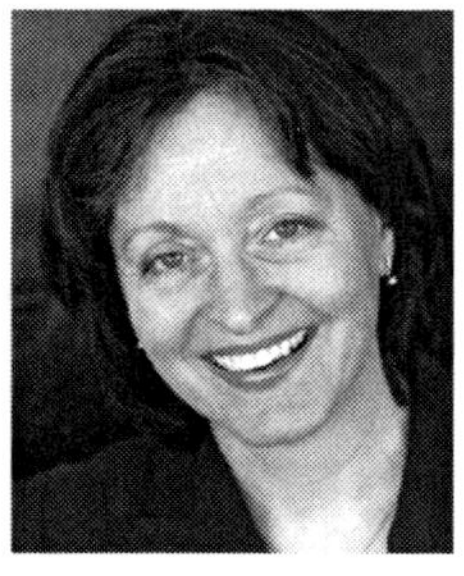

"My dream is that one day any patient who enters a hospital or doctor's office will have the choice of receiving procedure hypnosis to reduce stress and pain during the encounter and facilitate better medical outcomes."

Elvira Lang, MD, FSIR, FSCEH, is a pioneer and leading world expert in the use of hypnosis during medical procedures. Her research-based refinement of hypnotic techniques has resulted in greater patient comfort, increased practitioner effectiveness, and improved financial performance. Dr. Lang is Associate Professor of Radiology at Harvard Medical School and founder of Hypnalgesics, LLC, which trains medical teams in rapid rapport and quick hypnotic techniques. She is internationally known in the field of interventional radiology; she served as Chief of Interventional Radiology at the Beth Israel Deaconess Medical Center/Harvard Medical School in Boston from 1998 through 2006. Dr. Lang has trained nurses, doctors and technologists to incorporate procedure hypnosis into medical areas from a variety of disciplines including MRI, breast care, oncology, urology, gastroenterology, diagnostic and interventional radiology, obstetrics, and dentistry. She held faculty appointments and leadership positions at the University of Heidelberg, Stanford University, the University of Iowa Hospital and Clinics, and the Beth Israel Deaconess Medical Center. Dr. Lang takes an active leadership role in the advance of hypnosis in the medical setting; she is past president of the New England Society of Clinical Hypnosis, and current President of the Society of Clinical and Experimental Hypnosis.

PHOTO: JINSEY DAUK

Eleanor Laser

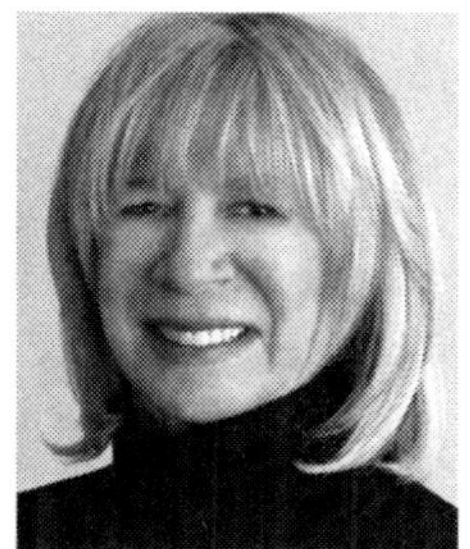

"As a professional hypnotherapist for 30 years, I am dedicated to promoting the hypnosis option for patients. Procedure hypnosis strengthens vital signs, reduces stress on practitioners and patients, and hastens recovery."

Eleanor Laser, PhD, is a clinical psychologist with extensive experience in using procedure hypnosis and hypnosis-assisted childbirth to ensure healthy patient outcomes. In addition to her private practice, she works in a number of medical settings. Dr. Laser is widely published, and lectures internationally. She has taught hypnosis techniques to psychologists and medical professionals around the world. Dr. Laser is an Approved Consultant for the American Society of Clinical Hypnosis (ASCH). She has served as trainer at the University of Iowa Hospital and Clinics in the Department of Interventional Radiology. At the Beth Israel Deaconess Medical Center, she partnered with Dr. Lang to develop training programs in rapid rapport and hypnosis adapted to the fast-paced nature of the modern patient encounter.

PHOTO: BOB HALL

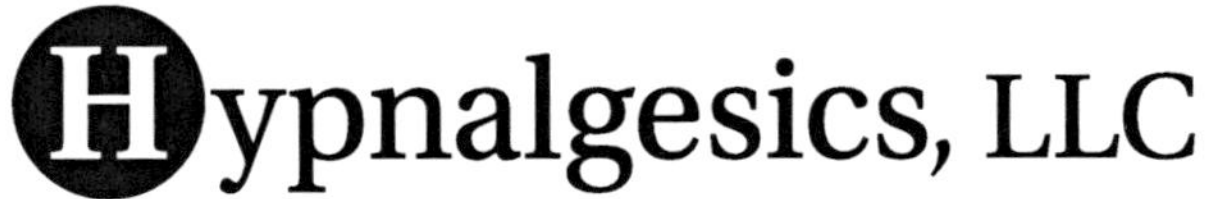

The Leading Voice in Patient Comfort

Hypnalgesics, LLC designs and delivers training in procedure hypnosis, rapid rapport and quick hypnotic techniques for greater patient comfort, practitioner effectiveness, and improved financial performance.

We serve hospitals, private practices, individuals, emergency rooms, MRI facilities, breast centers, surgical units, childbirth facilities, dental practices, chiropractic offices, radiology departments, and others.

Patient Sedation Without Medication **Bonus Chapter**. To download a bonus chapter that summarizes an actual procedure hypnosis experience from the point of view of both the practitioner and the patient, please visit **www.hypnalgesics.com/bonuschapter**

If you would like to receive our special report on the use of procedure hypnosis on practice effectiveness please contact us at **www.hypnalgesics.com/report**

To request a free initial evaluation of your facility visit us online at **www.hypnalgesics.com/evaluation**

Dr. Lang may be reached at **info@hypnalgesics.com**

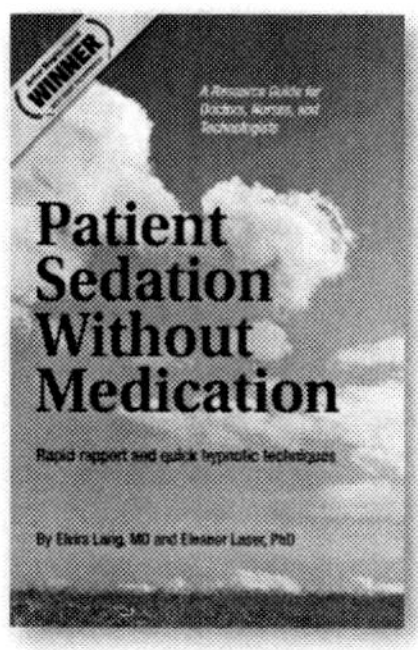

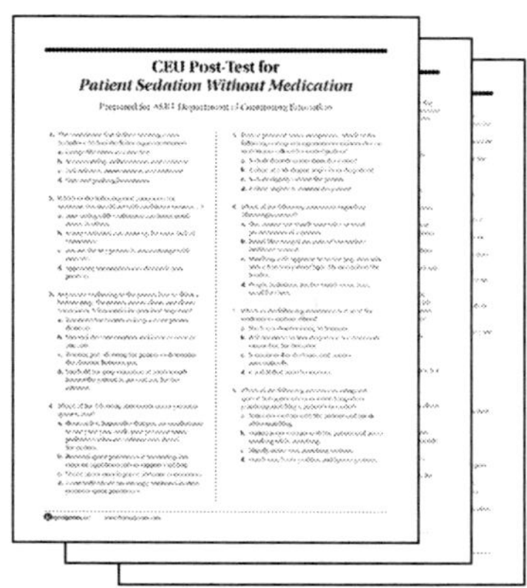
CEU Post-Test for
Patient Sedation Without Medication

Patient Sedation Without Medication is an ASRT APPROVED Category A+ Continuing Education Self-Learning Activity for Radiologic Technologists and Radiologist Assistants.

The American Society of Radiologic Technologists (ASRT) will award **9 A+ continuing education units (CEUs)** to Radiologic Technologists and Radiologist Assistants who read the text and achieve a passing score on the corresponding post-test of *Patient Sedation Without Medication: Rapid rapport and quick hypnotic techniques. A Resource Guide for Doctors, Nurses, and Technologists [E. Lang, MD and E. Laser PhD].* The cost of this A+ category 9 CEU activity is $80.00. Complete information, registration, and the post-test are available at **http://www.hypnalgesics.com/pages/CEU.html**

CPSIA information can be obtained at www.ICGtesting.com
Printed in the USA
LVOW091632200712

290925LV00009B/154/P

9 781461 037606